*American Diabetes
Association
Holiday Cookbook*

American Diabetes Association Holiday Cookbook

Betty Wedman, M.S., R.D.

Prentice Hall Press • *New York*

Published by Prentice Hall Press
A Division of Simon & Schuster, Inc.
Gulf + Western Building
One Gulf + Western Plaza
New York, NY 10023

PRENTICE HALL PRESS is a trademark of Simon & Schuster, Inc.

Library of Congress Cataloging-in-Publication Data

Wedman, Betty.
   American Diabetes Association holiday cookbook.

   Includes index.
   1. Diabetes—Diet therapy—Recipes.   2. Holiday
cookery.   I. American Diabetes Association.   II. Title.
RC662.W36   1986   641.5′6314   86-12247
ISBN 0-13-024894-0

Manufactured in the United States of America

10   9   8   7   6   5   4   3   2   1

First Edition

To

My mother, Betty St. Louis, who taught me how to cook and bake at the early age of seven. She was amazed at how many dishes I could dirty in making just one pan of brownies.

And to

Dorothy and Elsie Irvine of Hinsdale, Illinois, who worked diligently in typing and proofreading my original manuscript. They often served as taste-testers for many of the baked foods. Through the efforts of Dorothy and her eighty-year-old mother, Elsie, I was able to produce a quality cookbook with kitchen-tested recipes that are accurately written for your culinary delight.

Acknowledgments

Writing a book takes the dedicated efforts of many people. I am indebted to the American Diabetes Association and Carolyn Stevens, in particular, for believing in the need for a holiday cookbook and devoting so much effort in assisting with the publisher, Prentice Hall Press. I am also indebted to Sue Coughlin and the ADA reviewers: Melinda Downie Maryniuk, R.D., Carolyn Towers, R.D., and Debbie Hinnen, R.N. are to be commended for their hours of effort in laboring over the recipes for corrections and errors before the first copies rolled off the press.

A special thanks to my publisher Prentice Hall Press for the opportunity to share these recipes and menus with you. Through their special efforts I was able to provide you with these holiday goodies.

Contents

Foreword   xi

Introduction   xiii

1   Nutrition Basics   1

2   Adjusting Your Favorite Recipes   9

3   Holiday Menus   17

4   Festive Appetizers and Beverages   27

5   Yummy Salads and Soups   47

6   Vegetables and Fruits to Add Menu Glamour   69

7   Stuffings, Dressings, and Casseroles   83

8   Aromatic Yeast Breads and Coffee Cakes   101

9   Holiday Desserts   121

10   Tempting Muffins and Quick Breads   131

11   Special Cakes   149

12   Turkey Recipes for Leftovers   155

13   Traditional Jewish Recipes   173

14   Meal Planning and Food Exchanges   189

Appendix A   207

Appendix B   209

Index   211

Foreword

Holidays just naturally conjure up images of good things to eat—from a freshly roasted Thanksgiving turkey to Passover's challah and gefilte fish. No matter what our cultural or religious heritage, holiday food plays an important part in our traditional celebrations.

People with diabetes need not be deprived of the pleasures that holiday cooking can bring. If you or a member of your family has diabetes, you may need to control calories carefully, strictly limit sugar, and reduce salt, fat, and cholesterol in your diet. But you can still enjoy traditional holiday meals without abandoning the basics of good nutrition or prudent meal planning.

The *American Diabetes Association Holiday Cookbook* offers a wide array of recipes for holiday meals that will tempt the entire family. A quick glance through its pages will convince you that healthy eating and holiday celebrations are not mutually exclusive.

As the nation's largest voluntary health organization concerned with diabetes, the American Diabetes Association (ADA) is dedicated to improving the well-being of all people with diabetes and their families. Equally important is our unceasing support for research to find a preventive and cure for this chronic disease that affects some 11 million Americans.

The ADA carries out this important mission through the efforts of thousands of volunteers working at affiliates and chapters in more than 800 communities throughout the United States.

Membership in the ADA puts you in contact with a network of more than 225,000 caring people. Our local affiliates and chapters offer support groups, educational programs, counseling, and other special services. Membership in the ADA also brings with it twelve issues of our lively patient magazine, *Diabetes Forecast*. Each issue is packed with practical information on diabetes management.

The ADA also distributes a free quarterly newsletter with practical advice and helpful hints on living with diabetes.

Information on ADA membership and programs is available through our state affiliates, listed in the white pages of the telephone directory, or through the American Diabetes Association₍ₐ₎, Inc., Diabetes Information Service Center®, 1660 Duke Street, Alexandria, Virginia 22314, 800-ADA-DISC. (In Virginia and the Washington, DC metro area, dial 703-549-1500.)

We hope you enjoy the *American Diabetes Association Holiday Cookbook*. We think the book provides a wonderful way to celebrate your favorite holidays and celebrate good health, too. Bon appétit!

—AMERICAN DIABETES ASSOCIATION

Introduction

This book was written in response to requests from many people who receive diabetes counseling at the Hinsdale Medical Center in Hinsdale, Illinois. Most of the recipes were first introduced at an annual workshop on holiday cooking held at the center each fall.

The recipes have been carefully adjusted to be low in sugar, fat, and salt, yet tasty and easy to make. Like most cooks, I don't like being a slave to the kitchen, so my goal was to develop simple recipes that produce top-quality results.

I devoted many hours to a computer analysis of the nutrient values of each recipe. Exchange equivalents, newly revised for the first time in ten years to reflect the latest scientific findings on good nutrition and healthy eating, have been calculated for single servings of each recipe. They are based on the new *Exchange Lists for Meal Planning,* which are distributed by the American Diabetes Association and the American Dietetic Association.

The exchanges are listed with the recipe to help you adapt a given recipe to your own meal plan. The number of calories and grams of protein, fat, and carbohydrate per serving are also listed, along with milligrams of sodium and potassium, and cholesterol content.

As a past president of the American Association of Diabetes Educators and an active member of the American Diabetes Association, I know only too well the importance of good nutrition in diabetes care. People with diabetes need to realize that most foods can be included in a meal plan. Quantity—or portion size—is the key factor to be controlled.

Enjoy these holiday foods in moderation, and you, too, can partake of the great bounty that marks our holiday celebrations.

—BETTY WEDMAN, M.S., R.D.

American Diabetes Association Association Holiday Cookbook

1
NUTRITION BASICS

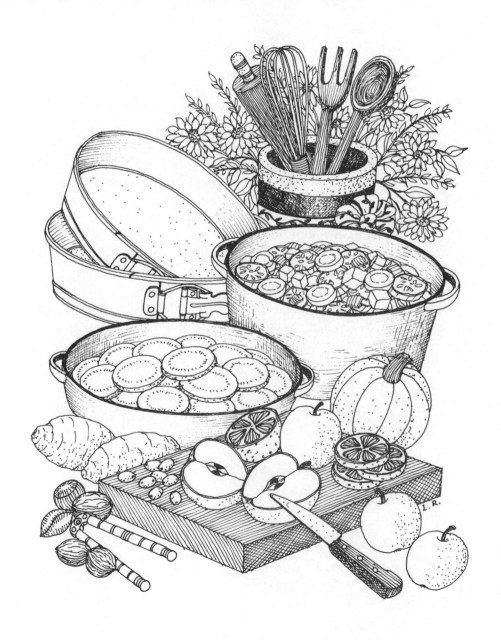

There are many recipes, especially in chapters 4 and 5, that require the use of a low-calorie sweetener. Although other low-calorie sweeteners can be used, the author suggests using Equal®, the brand name for the low-calorie sweetener aspartame. Equal does not leave an aftertaste as do other sweeteners that contain saccharin.

The Basics

Good nutrition is essential for good health. The principles of good nutrition are the same for everyone.

The following seven basic nutritional guidelines were designed by experts for the federal government to promote healthful eating and to reduce the risk of food-related diseases in the general population. They are also consistent with currently recommended principles for the nutritional management of diabetes. They are appropriate for the whole family—small children and adolescents, as well as adults.

1. Eat a variety of foods. There are up to fifty known nutrients that the body needs to stay healthy, and no single food contains them all. The wider the variety of foods in your diet, the less likely you are to develop either a deficiency or an excess of any single nutrient. Variety also reduces the likelihood of exposure to large amounts of contaminants in any single food.

It is important to choose foods from each of the four major food groups—milk and milk products, fruits and vegetables, breads, and meats—to ensure variety in your daily diet. However, it's just as important to vary the foods *within* each of the food groups.

2. Adjust calorie intake and exercise for proper weight. Calories are the basic units of measurement of energy taken in and used up by the body. When the food you eat provides more calories than your body needs, unused calories are converted to fat—the body's main storage depot for energy—and you gain weight.

To lose one pound of body fat, you must cut 3,500 calories from your food intake. Exercise of any kind will also help to use up the calories. It also may be beneficial to reduce your intake of fat. The body gets its energy (calories) from four sources: protein, carbohydrate, fat, and alcohol. Measure for measure, fat contains about twice as many calories as carbohydrate or protein. That's why fat has to be monitored even more carefully than the other calorie suppliers when you are trying to lose weight.

3. Limit fats and consumption of high-fat foods. Fatty foods pose more than just a weight-control problem. Excess fat—particularly saturated fats and cholesterol—may contribute to heart disease. Certain kinds of cancer may also be linked to fat intake. The average American gets 40 to 50 percent of his or her total calories from foods high in fat. Most dietitians recommend that adults reduce fat consumption to 30 to 35 percent of total calorie intake.

Fat consumption can be reduced by making informed food choices, eating smaller portions, trimming fat before cooking, cooking with lowfat methods, and eating more dried peas and beans, grain products, fruits, vegetables, low-fat dairy products, and low-fat meats.

4. Increase intake of unrefined carbohydrates and limit intake of refined carbohydrates. Gram for gram, all carbohydrates contain the same number of calories, but different sources of carbohydrates vary in overall nutritional value.

Biochemically, carbohydrates are subdivided into three groups. The term "sugar" or "simple" carbohydrate is usually applied to "monosaccharides" (which have one sugar group per molecule) and "disaccharides" (which have two sugar groups per molecule). The term "complex" carbohydrate usually refers to "polysaccharides," which have many sugar groups per molecule.

Complex carbohydrates are found primarily in legumes (beans and peas), grain products, and vegetables. Simple carbohydrates are found naturally in fruit and milk. These foods are each important sources of many essential nutrients, such as vitamins, minerals, and fiber.

However, when carbohydrates are processed or "refined" into commercial sugar and other sweeteners, they are left with calories but very little else in the way of nutritional value. That's why calories in refined carbohydrates are often called "empty" or "naked."

5. Increase consumption of fiber-rich foods. Fiber, or roughage, is the portion of plants that the human body cannot readily digest. Rich sources of fiber include complex or unrefined carbohydrates, such as fresh vegetables and fruits, whole grains, beans, peas, and nuts.

6. Reduce intake of sodium. Sodium, like saturated fat, may be associated with health problems, notably high blood pressure. The primary source of sodium in the American diet is table salt, which is about 40 percent sodium. (One teaspoon of salt weighs 5 grams and has about 2,000 milligrams of sodium.)

Relatively large amounts of sodium also enter our diet through convenience foods of all kinds. Foods that are salty to the taste—bacon or pickles, for example—may well contain high levels of sodium. Taste alone is not always an accurate indicator, however. Commercial soups, peanut butters, and salad dressings are a few of the many common foods that frequently have substantial amounts of sodium.

Food manufacturers commonly print the sodium content of their products on the package label. In addition, several food companies have developed tasty, low-sodium lines. However, many canned goods still contain high sodium levels, so it is a good idea to rinse these foods under tap water for a full minute before cooking or serving.

7. Use alcohol sparingly, if at all. Alcohol is high in calories and has almost no nutritional value. Therefore, if weight reduction is an issue, even light drinkers should consider cutting back on those empty calories.

The general rule: If you do drink, do so in moderation at all times. One or two drinks daily appear to cause no harm in most adults. Pregnant women, however, should avoid alcohol to be on the safe side. People with diabetes should consult their physicians about alcohol use; they may have to observe special restrictions concerning times for drinking and amounts consumed.

Nutrition and Diabetes

T he dietary recommendations of the American Diabetes Association are similar to the general nutritional guidelines outlined above. However, they take into account the special concerns of people who have diabetes.

Diabetes is a disorder characterized by the body's failure properly to convert glucose—the fuel derived from food—into energy for the body's cells. Insulin, a hormone produced in the pancreas, helps body cells use blood glucose (sugar). If the body produces no insulin or is unable to use the insulin properly, the result is high levels of glucose in the blood. High blood-glucose levels can cause immediate problems, such as fatigue and excessive hunger, thirst and frequent urination, as well as long-term complications.

Diabetes has two major forms: (a) type I (insulin-dependent) diabetes and (b) type II (non-insulin-dependent) diabetes. Diet plays an important part in the control of both.

People with type I diabetes produce essentially no insulin. As a result, they need daily injections of insulin to survive. Insulin lowers blood-glucose levels and would cause *low* blood glucose if the user did not eat enough food. Therefore, people with type I diabetes have to eat enough food to avoid low blood glucose, but not so much as to overcome the insulin and send blood glucose soaring. This is quite a balancing act, because food and insulin are not the only factors that affect blood-glucose levels. Exercise, for instance, generally lowers blood glucose, and stress (either emotional or physical) can raise it. About 10 percent of people with diabetes have this form of the disease, which usually appears in people under the age of thirty.

People with type II diabetes can produce insulin. In fact, they may have a normal or even higher-than-normal amount. However, the insulin is not as effective as it should be, a problem known as insulin resistance. Insulin resistance is largely due to excess body fat, which is common in people with type II diabetes. This form of diabetes usually develops after age forty.

About 90 percent of people with diabetes have non-insulin-dependent diabetes, and about 80 percent of them are overweight at the time of diagnosis. Being too fat seems to make people resistant to insulin, whether or not they have diabetes. Losing weight often causes a remarkable improvement. Therefore, weight loss and maintenance of ideal weight is a major goal of therapy in overweight patients with type II diabetes. Exercise also helps the body to use its insulin and to lower blood-glucose levels, so most doctors recommend a combination of caloric limitation and regular exercise.

Some people with type II diabetes take insulin or pills for controlling blood glucose when their weight loss and exercise programs do not do the job. People who are treated with insulin, and some people who are treated with pills, need to eat food at prescribed times. But those whose diabetes is managed by diet and exercise alone are not prone to low blood glucose. Therefore, it is not as important for them to eat on a rigid schedule.

A small number of people with type II diabetes are of normal or near-normal weight when they develop the condition. These people, too, can often benefit from losing a few pounds, especially if they are pushing the high end of normal. However, not everyone needs to reduce.

If you are relatively thin and have type II diabetes, you may find that frequent small feedings are better than three big meals a day. Smaller meals allow the body to use its insulin most efficiently, because they do not make heavy demands on the pancreas for insulin. Fiber-rich and whole foods, as well as regular exercise, are also recommended to help reduce blood-glucose fluctuation.

No matter what kind of diabetes you have, the following are the goals of diet therapy:

- Improve overall health through optimal nutrition.
- Provide for normal growth in children.
- Achieve and/or maintain a body weight appropriate for height.
- Maintain blood glucose at as close to normal levels as possible.
- Prevent or delay heart, kidney, eye, nerve, and other complications associated with diabetes. (Much research suggests that keeping blood-glucose levels at or near the normal range may prevent or delay long-term complications.)

To achieve these goals, the American Diabetes Association recommends the following guidelines, in addition to the nutritional guidelines outlined above.

• Pay particular attention to caloric intake. Excess calories cause high blood-glucose levels and obesity.
• Strictly limit your intake of *refined* carbohydrates (sugars). In addition to being low in vitamins and other nutrients, these sugary foods cause a rapid and high rise in blood glucose.
• Follow an individualized meal plan that suits your lifestyle. Work with a dietitian familiar with diabetes to develop the plan. Generally dietitians will suggest a meal plan in which about 50 to 60 percent of calories come from carbohydrate, mostly unrefined (dried beans and peas, whole-grain cereals and breads, vegetables, fruit); 12 to 20 percent from protein; and the rest from fat, mainly vegetable fat. Many dietitians also recommend that you follow a meal plan based on the *Exchange Lists for Meal Planning*, a publication of the American Diabetes Association and the American Dietetic Association. (See chapter 14 for a description of the exchange lists.)

Holiday Cooking and Indulging

Holidays are fun for everyone. People with diabetes, too, can have holiday favorites like fruitcake, Christmas stollen, and cranberry orange muffins by making them from the simple recipes given in this cookbook. When you add these treats to your diet, be sure to make the appropriate substitutions in your meal plan.

All the holiday favorites represented in this book have been specially designed to be low in fat, salt, and sugar. In addition, the recipes conform to the American Diabetes Association's guideline of no more than one-half teaspoon of sugar per serving. (The only exceptions to this rule are the Honey Cake, page 184, the Zimsterne, page 177, and the Mandelbrot, page 182. Slightly more sugar was used to preserve the traditional character of these recipes.)

People with diabetes *can* enjoy these holiday treats, as long as they are carefully worked into the individual meal plan. Holiday eating does require some self-discipline, though. Don't be fooled into thinking that you can consume large quantities of these foods just because they are low in sugar and fat. One or two cookies can be incorporated into a meal plan as a special treat. Four cookies or an extra piece of pie can wreak havoc with your diabetes control.

Let moderation be your guide. When friends raise their eyebrows and ask, "Can you eat that?", you can smile and say "Yes" proudly. You know that you have carefully planned your day's meals to include some holiday treats. Better still, you can tell your friends that your selection of goodies is healthier for them because it contains less fat, salt, and sugar than conventional recipes or supermarket products. Before long, you may find them following your lead to a more nutritious diet.

2

Adjusting Your Favorite Recipes

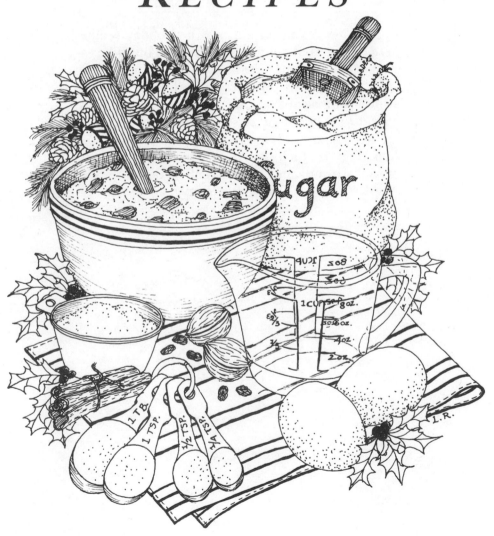

Do you have a favorite holiday recipe that you want to prepare but it has a cup of sugar or two cups of butter? Read this section and learn how to adjust your recipe so that it will offer more nutrition with less sugar, less salt, and less fat.

Note: For the purposes of this book, all temperatures are indicated in Fahrenheit degrees. See Appendix B for Centigrade conversions.

Many recipes in use today do not have the low-sugar, lowfat, low-sodium, and high-fiber content of those presented in this book. The time has come to look closely at your recipes and be sure that they provide good nutrition and stay within accepted dietary guidelines.

You can begin to adjust your family's favorite recipes by using the basic proportions presented in this chapter. Start by comparing your recipe with the nutritious recipe to see where modifications can be made. Reducing the **salt** or omitting it completely is the least noticeable change (except in yeast breads where salt is used to control yeast growth). **Sugar** is next on the list. In many cases, your family will hardly notice that you have cut the sugar content in their chocolate chip cookies. The cookies will just be less crisp and not spread out on the pan quite as far. Modifying **fat** content, by reducing margarine, butter, or shortening, can be a little more tricky. Extra moisture may be needed in the form of water, skim milk, or an extra egg.

Here are several examples of how recipes can be adjusted to yield a more nutritious product. You may think the nutrition comparison charts are not significant enough to warrant your changing the ingredients. Take another look at the *percentage* figures and you will see why the modifications are important to produce a more nutritional food.

PEANUT BUTTER COOKIES
(Makes 36 cookies)

Original Recipe

½ cup shortening
½ cup peanut butter,
  smooth or chunky
½ cup granulated sugar
½ cup brown sugar
1 egg
1¼ cups flour
½ teaspoon baking
  powder
¾ teaspoon baking soda
¼ teaspoon salt

Nutritious Recipe

¼ cup vegetable oil
½ cup peanut butter,
  smooth or chunky
½ cup light or dark
  brown sugar
1 egg
1¼ cups flour
½ teaspoon baking
  powder
¾ teaspoon baking
  soda
No salt needed
¼ cup water

*M*ix the shortening (oil), peanut butter, sugar, and egg together. Stir in the remaining ingredients. Chill the dough for 3 hours or overnight. Roll into walnut-sized balls. Place on a lightly oiled baking sheet. Flatten with a fork. Bake in a 375-degree oven for 10 to 12 minutes. Cool thoroughly before serving.

Nutrition Comparison

	Original	Nutritious Recipe
Calories per cookie	85	61
Protein	1.5 g	1.5 g
Carbohydrate	9 g	6.4 g
Fat	5 g	3.5 g
Sodium	58 mg	44 mg
Cholesterol	8 mg	8 mg

Nutrient Percentage Comparison

	Original	Nutritious Recipe
Protein	7%	10%
Carbohydrate	41	40
Fat	52	50*

* The fat content is lower in saturated fats than the original recipe because oil was used instead of shortening.

The original recipe for Peanut Butter Cookies has twice the fat and sugar content as the nutritious recipe. Baking powder and baking soda both add sodium so salt is not needed for flavoring. Water is added to the nutritious recipe to give a moist texture because the fat content has been reduced. *There are 28 percent fewer calories and 24 percent less sodium in the nutritious recipe.*

Here are the basic proportions for cookies. Higher fat and sugar content is what makes a drop cookie spread. Nuts, coconut, and sunflower seeds add to the fat content so keep the quantity used to limited amounts.

1 cup flour
½ cup sugar, honey, or molasses (dark or light)
0 to ⅛ teaspoon salt (optional)
2 to 3 tablespoons margarine, butter, shortening, or oil
1 egg
¼ to ½ cup lowfat milk
1 to 2 teaspoons baking powder

Muffins

Muffins are another food where adjustments can easily be made in recipes to show improved nutritional content. They need only enough sweetness to complement the other ingredients in the batter, like corn, bran, raisins, or blueberries. Salt is not needed because the baking powder and baking soda add a significant amount of sodium for flavor. Vegetable oil is preferred as the fat to provide increased polyunsaturated fats in the diet.

B L U E B E R R Y   M U F F I N S

(Makes 16)

Original Recipe

3 cups flour
1½ teaspoons salt
4½ teaspoons baking
   powder
5 tablespoons sugar
2 eggs
1½ cups milk
½ cup shortening, melted
1 cup blueberries

Nutritious Recipe

3 cups whole wheat
   flour
No salt needed
4½ teaspoons baking
   powder
3 tablespoons sugar
1 egg
1 egg white
1½ cups milk
3 tablespoons vegetable
   oil
1 cup blueberries

Combine the flour, baking powder, and sugar in a bowl. Add the egg, egg white, milk, and oil (melted shortening). Stir just until the ingredients are moistened. Gently fold in the blueberries. Spoon into lightly oiled muffin tins. Bake in a 425-degree oven for 20 to 25 minutes.

Nutrition Comparison

	Original	Nutritious Recipe
Calories per serving	182	128
Protein	4 g	4 g
Carbohydrate	23 g	21 g
Fat	8 g	4 g
Sodium	274 mg	90 mg
Cholesterol	38 mg	18 mg

Nutrient Percentage Comparison

	Original	Nutritious Recipe
Protein	9%	13%
Carbohydrate	51	65
Fat	40	28*

* The fat content is lower in saturated fats than the original recipe because oil was used instead of melted shortening.

The original recipe for Blueberry Muffins has been reduced in sugar, salt, and fat content. One egg plus an egg white were used to lower cholesterol. Two egg whites could have been used instead of the 2 eggs if a very low cholesterol diet is followed. *The nutritious recipe has 67 percent less sodium and 53 percent less cholesterol* plus the lower fat and sugar content.

Here are the basic proportions for making a nutritious muffin. Compare your recipes to these levels and make adjustments accordingly.

1 cup flour
1 tablespoon sugar, honey, or molasses (dark or light)
0 to ⅛ teaspoon salt (optional)
1 tablespoon vegetable oil, margarine, butter, or
    shortening
½ egg
½ cup lowfat milk or liquid
1 to 2 teaspoons baking powder

Pancakes

Pancakes are similar to muffins in basic recipe proportions. A pancake batter has more liquid than a muffin. The higher amounts of sugar used in muffins helps tenderize the batter so a fine even texture is formed in baking. Pancakes cook very fast so only a small amount of sugar is needed to tenderize the product.

BUTTERMILK PANCAKES

(Makes sixteen 4-inch pancakes)

Original Recipe

1 egg
1¼ cups buttermilk
2 tablespoons margarine,
   melted
1¼ cups flour
1 tablespoon sugar
1 teaspoon baking powder
½ teaspoon baking soda
½ teaspoon salt

Nutritious Recipe

1 egg white
1¼ cups buttermilk
1 tablespoon vegetable oil
1¼ cups flour
1 teaspoon sugar
1 teaspoon baking powder
½ teaspoon baking soda
No salt needed

*B*eat the egg, buttermilk, and oil (melted margarine) together. Add the flour, sugar, baking powder, and baking soda. Stir just until all the ingredients are mixed. Pour the batter onto a lightly oiled griddle. Cook until bubbles form on the surface and edges become dry. Turn; cook 2 minutes longer, or until browned.

Nutrition Comparison

	Original	Nutritious Recipe
Calories per pancake	61	50
Protein	2 g	2 g
Carbohydrate	9 g	8 g
Fat	2 g	1 g
Sodium	143 mg	64 mg
Cholesterol	18 mg	1 mg

Nutrient Percentage Comparison

	Original	Nutritious Recipe
Protein	12%	17%
Carbohydrate	59	64
Fat	29	19

The original recipe for Buttermilk Pancakes has twice the fat and more than double the sugar and salt content as the nutritious recipe. Vegetable oil was used to give a high polyunsaturated fat content and salt was omitted because baking powder, baking soda, and buttermilk all contain sodium. *There is 55 percent less sodium in the nutritious recipe and 94 percent less cholesterol,* in addition to less fat and more protein per calorie in the nutritious Buttermilk Pancake recipe.

Here are the basic proportions for pancakes. To use whole wheat flour, substitute half the flour in the recipe with whole wheat.

1 cup flour
0 to 1 teaspoon sugar, honey, or molasses (dark or
  light)
0 to ⅛ teaspoon salt (optional)
2 teaspoons vegetable oil, margarine, or butter
½ egg
¾ to 1 cup lowfat milk or liquid
1 to 2 teaspoons baking powder

3

HOLIDAY MENUS

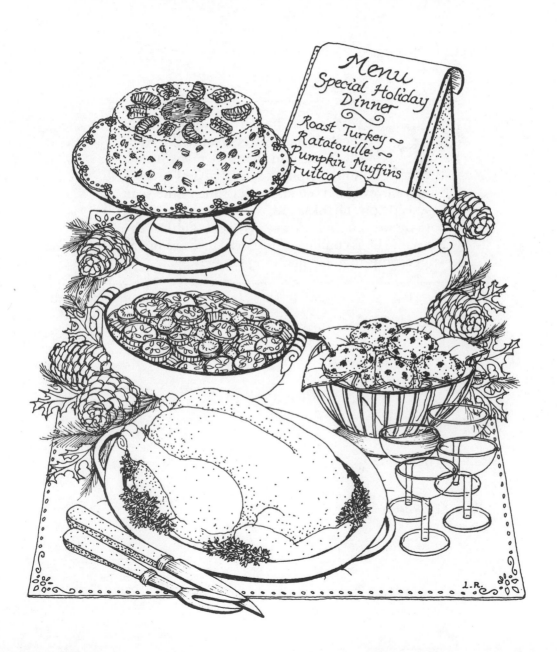

Menu
Special Holiday
Dinner

Roast Turkey ~
Ratatouille ~
Pumpkin Muffins
Fruitca...

*E*very meal has a menu. Holiday meals usually offer a wide selection of foods and feature many traditional family treats. Brussels sprouts might never be served any other time of the year —except on Thanksgiving, when everyone enjoys them with their turkey. What about the vegetarian who is coming to dinner? Here are menu suggestions to make planning easier.

Thanksgiving Breakfast
Fresh Fruit Ambrosia
Pumpkin Pancakes with Rum Sauce
Beverage

Thanksgiving Dinner
Spicy Tomato Cocktail
Potato Hors d'Oeuvres   Salmon Dip
Roast Turkey and Apricot Dressing
Cranapple Relish
Brussels Sprouts with Walnuts   Sweet Potatoes à l'Orange
Traditional Waldorf Salad
Pumpkin–Bran Muffins   Banana Bread
Beverage

Thanksgiving Night Snack
Purée of Broccoli Soup
Cheese and Crackers
Pumpkin Fruitcake
Beverage

Thanksgiving Dinner for 2 or 4
Broiled Mushroom Caps
Baked Cornish Hens with Cranberry–Wild Rice Stuffing
Vegetable Confetti
Orange Waldorf Salad
Pumpkin–Raisin Muffins
Beverage

Lacto-Ovo Vegetarian Thanksgiving Dinner
(milk, egg, and cheese are eaten)
Spicy Tomato Cocktail
Potato Hors d'Oeuvres   Moroccan Dip
Cheese and Rice Casserole
Brussels Sprouts with Walnuts   Sweet Potatoes à l'Orange
Traditional Waldorf Salad
Pumpkin–Bran Muffins   Banana Bread

Lacto-Ovo Vegetarian Thanksgiving Night Snack
Purée of Broccoli Soup
Cheese and Crackers
Pumpkin Fruitcake
Beverage

All-Vegetable Vegetarian Thanksgiving Dinner
(no animal products are eaten)
Spicy Tomato Cocktail
Vegetable–Barley Soup
Rice and Lentils   Apple and Prune Dressing
Brussels Sprouts with Walnuts   Sweet Potatoes à l'Orange
Traditional Waldorf Salad
Pumpkin–Bran Muffins*   Banana Bread*
Beverage

All-Vegetable Vegetarian Thanksgiving Night Snack
(no animal products are eaten)
Purée of Broccoli Soup
Four-Bean Salad   Whole Wheat Toast
Pumpkin Fruitcake
Beverage

* Orange or apple juice can be used to replace milk in recipe. Egg can be omitted or 1 tablespoon arrowroot or cornstarch substituted per egg.

Christmas Eve Midnight Supper
Hot Wassail
Broiled Herbed Scallops   Baked Shrimp Scampi
Pears with Ricotta
Fruitcake
Assorted Cookies
Beverage

Christmas Brunch
Christmas Cranberry Punch
Brunch Pizza
Holiday Cranberry Rolls
Sliced Oranges and Kiwi
Beverage

Christmas Dinner
Low-Calorie Eggnog   Merry Cranberry Punch
Cherry Tomatoes with Pesto Filling   Oysters Casino
Roast Turkey with Corn Bread Stuffing
Baked Pumpkin   Cauliflower Piquante
Sliced Beet Salad
Christmas Stollen   Cranberry–Orange Muffins
Assorted Cookies
Beverage

Lacto-Ovo Vegetarian Christmas Eve Midnight Supper
(milk, egg, and cheese are eaten)
Hot Wassail
Pears with Ricotta   Carrot–Cottage Cheese Dip
Fruitcake   Assorted Cookies
Beverage

Lacto-Ovo Vegetarian Christmas Brunch
(milk, egg, and cheese are eaten)
Christmas Cranberry Punch
Scrambled Eggs   Holiday Cranberry Rolls
Sliced Oranges and Kiwi
Beverage

Lacto-Ovo Vegetarian Christmas Dinner
(milk, egg, and cheese are eaten)
Low-Calorie Eggnog
Cherry Tomatoes with Pesto Filling
Eggplant–Swiss Cheese Casserole   Traditional Bread Dressing
Baked Pumpkin   Cauliflower Piquante
Sliced Beet Salad
Christmas Stollen   Cranberry–Orange Muffins
Assorted Cookies
Beverage

All-Vegetable Vegetarian Christmas Midnight Supper
(no animal products are eaten)
Hot Wassail
Hearty Lentil Soup
Fruitcake   Assorted Cookies
Beverage

All-Vegetable Vegetarian Christmas Brunch
(no animal products are eaten)
Christmas Cranberry Punch
Gingerbread Waffle*
Fruit Sauce for Pancakes and Waffles
Beverage

* Orange or apple juice can be used to replace milk in recipe. Egg can be omitted or 1 tablespoon arrowroot or cornstarch substituted per egg.

All-Vegetable Vegetarian Christmas Dinner
(no animal products are eaten)
Merry Cranberry Punch
Tofu Fiesta   Traditional Bread Dressing
Baked Pumpkin   Cauliflower Piquante
Sliced Beet Salad
Christmas Stollen   Cranberry–Orange Muffins*
Assorted Cookies
Beverage

New Year's Eve Dinner
Fruit Punch
Oyster Stew
Broiled Swordfish
Wild Rice-Stuffed Squash
Broccoli Spears
Oatmeal–Banana Muffins
Beverage

New Year's Brunch
Raspberry Smoothie
Ricotta Cassata
Swedish Tea Log   Bran Muffins
Melon Wedge
Beverage

New Year's Supper
Stuffed Cheese Pizza
Beverage

* Orange or apple juice can be used to replace milk in recipe. Egg can be omitted or 1 tablespoon arrowroot or cornstarch substituted per egg.

Lacto-Ovo Vegetarian New Year's Eve Dinner
(milk, egg, and cheese are eaten)
Fruit Punch
Savory Potato Soup
Wild Rice-Stuffed Squash   Broccoli Spears
Oatmeal–Banana Muffins
Beverage

Lacto-Ovo New Year's Brunch
(milk, egg, and cheese are eaten)
Raspberry Smoothie
Ricotta Cassata
Swedish Tea Log   Bran Muffins
Melon Wedge
Beverage

Lacto-Ovo New Year's Supper
(milk, egg, and cheese are eaten)
Stuffed Cheese Pizza
Beverage

All-Vegetable Vegetarian New Year's Eve Dinner
(no animal products are eaten)
Fruit Punch
African Vegetarian Stew
Oatmeal–Banana Muffins
Assorted Cookies
Beverage

All-Vegetable Vegetarian New Year's Brunch
(no animal products are eaten)
Cranberry Cooler
Hearty Lentil Soup
Swedish Tea Log   Bran Muffins
Melon Wedge
Beverage

All-Vegetable Vegetarian New Year's Supper
(no animal products are eaten)
Whole Wheat Pizza
(substitute tofu for mozzarella cheese)
Beverage

Traditional Passover Seder Meal
Gefilte Fish with Horseradish
Chicken-Rice Soup
Roast Turkey
Sweet Potatoes à l'Orange
Cauliflower Piquante
Cranapple Relish
Dates and Figs

Rosh Hashanah Dinner
Fresh Sliced Pineapple
Lamb and Brown Rice Pilaf
Sweet and Sour Green Beans
Tzimmes
Challah
Mandelbrot   Zimsterne
Honey Cake

Sabbath Meal
Beef Cholent
Cucumber Salad   Dijon Broccoli Salad
Challah
Lokshen Kugel

4

FESTIVE APPETIZERS AND BEVERAGES

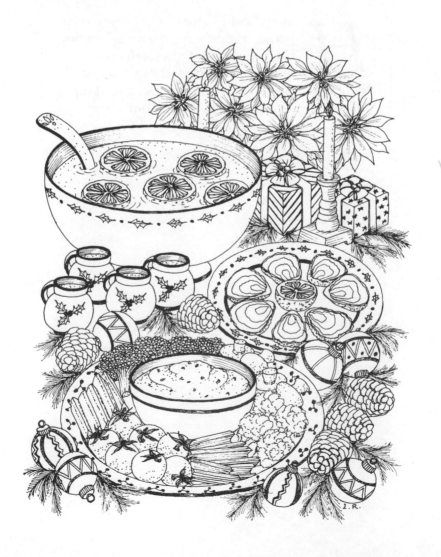

*H*ot and cold snacks help keep the appetite under control while waiting for other dinner guests to arrive. Indulge in some of these low-calorie dips, vegetable hors d'oeuvres, and beverages without sacrificing your diet and your appetite.

CHERRY TOMATOES WITH PESTO FILLING

(Serves 24)

24 cherry tomatoes
1 teaspoon dried basil
2 tablespoons pine nuts, toasted
1 small garlic clove, minced
1 ounce Parmesan cheese

*C*ut a small slice off the top of the tomatoes and hollow the tomatoes out. Put the tomatoes on a baking sheet. Combine the other ingredients in a blender or food processor. Blend until the cheese and nuts are ground. Stuff the mixture into the tomatoes. Refrigerate. Serve cold or heat in a 400-degree oven for 10 minutes before serving.

ONE SERVING
=
10 calories
1 CHO
0 PRO
0 FAT
9 SODIUM
64 POTASSIUM
0 CHOLESTEROL

Exchange Value:
FREE for 1 or 2
3 or 4 = 1 Vegetable
Exchange + 1/2 Fat
Exchange

SAPSAGO CHEESE ROLLS

(Serves 6)

18 Boston lettuce leaves
4 ounces lowfat ricotta cheese
3 ounces Sapsago cheese*, grated
¼ cup finely chopped walnuts
1 teaspoon prepared mustard OR ½ teaspoon
   powdered mustard
½ cup wine vinegar, red or white
¼ cup vegetable oil
1 teaspoon ground rosemary
1 head Boston lettuce
Minced fresh coriander or parsley leaves

*D*ip the lettuce leaves into boiling water and quickly plunge them into cold water. Drain off the water and trim off the vein in each leaf. Mix the cheeses and walnuts until well combined. Put a spoonful of the cheese mixture in the center of each leaf and roll up tightly. Place in a flat dish. Combine the remaining ingredients, except the coriander, and pour over the rolls. Cover the dish and refrigerate overnight, or at least 6 hours. Remove the rolls from the dressing. Serve at room temperature on a bed of Boston lettuce leaves. Sprinkle on the coriander. Extra dressing may be served with the rolls, if desired.

ONE SERVING
=
167 calories
4 CHO
5 PRO
13 FAT
34 SODIUM
208 POTASSIUM
11 CHOLESTEROL

Exchange Value:
1 Lean Meat
Exchange +
1 Vegetable Exchange
+ 2 Fat Exchanges

* If Sapsago cheese is not available, blue cheese may be substituted, but the fat content will be doubled.

SALMON DIP

(Makes 1½ cups)

1 7¾-ounce can salmon
2 tablespoons minced green onion (scallion)
¼ cup plain lowfat yogurt
¼ cup mayonnaise or salad dressing
½ teaspoon ground ginger
2 tablespoons sesame seeds, toasted
Raw vegetables: zucchini, celery, carrots, pea pods,
    cherry tomatoes

*D*rain and flake the salmon. Combine all the
ingredients, *except* the raw vegetables in a bowl. Cover
and refrigerate for at least 1 hour. Serve with the
vegetables.

ONE TABLESPOON
=
17 calories
0 CHO
0 PRO
1.5 FAT
106 SODIUM
16 POTASSIUM
1 CHOLESTEROL

Exchange Value:
1 tablespoon =
FREE
3 tablespoons =
1 Fat Exchange

MOROCCAN DIP

(Makes 1½ cups)

1 cup plain lowfat yogurt
½ cup part skim ricotta cheese
2 tablespoons chopped dried currants or dark or
    golden raisins
2 tablespoons chopped green onion (scallion)
1 small garlic clove, minced
½ teaspoon curry powder
⅛ teaspoon ground cinnamon

*C*ombine all the ingredients in bowl. Beat well. Cover
and chill for at least 1 hour to blend the flavors. Serve
with raw vegetables.

ONE TABLESPOON
=
17 calories
1 CHO
1 PRO
0 FAT
11 SODIUM
34 POTASSIUM
3 CHOLESTEROL

Exchange Value:
FREE

MARINATED CRAYFISH TAILS

(Serves 6)

2 pounds boiled crayfish tails
¾ cup olive oil
¾ cup cider vinegar
2 teaspoons celery seeds
Dash of Tabasco sauce
1 lemon, thinly sliced
1 small onion, thinly sliced

*P*eel the crayfish tails. Combine the other ingredients in a bowl and add the crayfish tails. Cover and marinate overnight or for at least 3 hours. Serve as appetizers or in a crayfish salad.

ONE SERVING
=

178 calories
3 CHO
11 PRO
12 FAT
1 SODIUM
103 POTASSIUM
90 CHOLESTEROL

Exchange Value:
1½ Lean Meat Exchanges + 2 Fat Exchanges

BARBECUED PRAWNS

(Serves 2)

1 pound prawns or unshelled jumbo shrimp
¼ cup barbecue sauce
2 tablespoons water

*R*emove the legs from the prawns or shrimp. Lay each on its side and cut about halfway through from the top of the shell. Marinate in a mixture of the barbecue sauce and water for 30 minutes. Cook on a grill or broil for 5 to 10 minutes, or until the shells are browned and the shrimp are pink.

ONE SERVING
=

104 calories
3 CHO
16 PRO
3 FAT
260 SODIUM
134 POTASSIUM
135 CHOLESTEROL

Exchange Value:
2 Lean Meat Exchanges

RICOTTA CASSATA

(Serves 8)

1¼ cups unbleached white flour
½ teaspoon salt
¼ cup margarine
3 to 4 tablespoons cold water
3 egg whites
1½ pounds ricotta cheese
¼ cup lowfat milk
¼ cup honey
1 teaspoon ground cinnamon

Make a crust by combining the flour, salt, and margarine in a bowl. Cut the margarine into the flour with a fork or pastry blender until crumbly. Sprinkle the water over the mixture. Toss with a fork until the pastry holds together. Place the dough on a lightly floured surface. Roll the dough into a large circle. Transfer to a 9-inch pie plate. Crimp the edges and trim.

Combine the egg whites, cheese, milk, and honey in a blender or food processor. Pour the mixture into the pastry shell. Sprinkle on the cinnamon. Bake in a 375-degree oven for 10 minutes. Lower the oven temperature to 350 degrees and bake for 25 to 30 minutes longer, or until a knife inserted into the center comes out clean. Cool slightly on a wire rack. Serve warm or cold.

ONE SERVING
=

291 calories
25 CHO
14 PRO
13 FAT
290 SODIUM
150 POTASSIUM
47 CHOLESTEROL

Exchange Value:
1 Bread Exchange +
1 Lean Meat
Exchange + ½ Milk
Exchange + 2 Fat
Exchanges

BROILED HERBED SCALLOPS

(Serves 2)

¼ pound fresh bay scallops
1 green onion (scallion), minced
2 tablespoons lemon juice
1 teaspoon vegetable oil
1 teaspoon dried basil
½ teaspoon dried tarragon
Chopped fresh parsley leaves

ONE SERVING
=
84 calories
0 CHO
13 PRO
3 FAT
150 SODIUM
275 POTASSIUM
30 CHOLESTEROL

Exchange Value:
2 Lean Meat
Exchanges

*P*ut the scallops in a bowl. Add the remaining ingredients, *except* the parsley. Toss and marinate at room temperature for 10 to 15 minutes. Remove the scallops from the marinade and put on wooden skewers or place in a shallow pan. Broil just until the scallops are opaque, being careful not to overcook. Baste with the marinade. Sprinkle on the parsley just before serving.

Note: Any leftover marinade may be refrigerated and used for halibut, salmon, and swordfish.

BAKED SHRIMP SCAMPI

(Serves 2)

½ pound unshelled raw fresh shrimp
1 tablespoon butter
1 small garlic clove, minced
1 teaspoon lemon juice
1 tablespoon chopped fresh parsley leaves
1 teaspoon grated Parmesan cheese

Wash the shrimp and remove the shells. Combine the butter, garlic, lemon juice, and parsley in a casserole. Bake in a 350-degree oven until the butter has melted. Arrange the shrimp over the butter sauce. Cover and bake for 10 to 12 minutes, or until the shrimp turn pink. Sprinkle on the cheese just before serving.

ONE SERVING
=

179 calories
0 CHO
16 PRO
12 FAT
149 SODIUM
85 POTASSIUM
136 CHOLESTEROL

Exchange Value:
2 Lean Meat Exchanges
+ 1 Fat Exchange

STEAMED MUSSELS

(Serves 2)

1 pound mussels
1 small garlic clove, minced
2 green onions (scallions), chopped
1 cup clam juice or dry white wine

Clean and rinse the mussels thoroughly. Combine the garlic, onions, and clam juice in a saucepan. Cook for 10 minutes to develop flavor. Add the mussels. Cover and cook over high heat until the mussels have opened. Immediately upon opening, the mussels should be removed from the broth. Serve as an appetizer.

ONE SERVING
=

65 calories
5 CHO
7 PRO
0 FAT
346 SODIUM
446 POTASSIUM
25 CHOLESTEROL

Exchange Value:
1 Lean Meat
Exchange

POTATO HORS D'OEUVRES

(Serves 18)

18 small red-skinned potatoes
½ pound fresh mushrooms
1 tablespoon dried dill
1 tablespoon dried parsley flakes
½ cup apple juice
1 teaspoon lemon juice
3 tablespoons grated Parmesan cheese

Wash the potatoes and steam them until they are fork-tender. Cut off a thin slice on the bottom of each potato to allow it to sit without rolling. Cut off a thin slice on top of each potato and scoop out the inside "meat" of the potato. Reserve the inside of the potato.

Poach the mushrooms in a saucepan with the dill, parsley flakes, apple juice, and lemon juice for 5 minutes. Pour off the liquid. Put the mushrooms and potato "meat" in a food processor or blender. Chop until fine. Stuff the potato skins with the mushroom filling. Sprinkle with the cheese. Refrigerate until ready to serve. When ready to serve, heat in a 350-degree oven for 15 to 20 minutes. Serve warm.

**ONE
SERVING**
=
*50 calories
10 CHO
2 PRO
0 FAT
18 SODIUM
204 POTASSIUM
1 CHOLESTEROL*

*Exchange Value:
1 Bread Exchange*

BROILED MUSHROOM CAPS
(Serves 4)

1 pound large fresh mushrooms
1 tablespoon margarine
1 tablespoon vegetable oil
2 tablespoons lemon juice
1 tablespoon grated Parmesan cheese

*R*emove the stems from the mushrooms and reserve for use in a meatloaf or omelet. Arrange the mushroom caps on a lightly oiled baking pan. Broil for 2 minutes. Turn over and broil 2 minutes more. Meanwhile, combine margarine, oil, and lemon juice in a saucepan or chafing dish. Pour over the mushrooms in a serving dish. Sprinkle on the Parmesan cheese and toss to blend.

ONE SERVING
=
71 calories
1 CHO
1 PRO
7 FAT
60 SODIUM
75 POTASSIUM
1 CHOLESTEROL

Exchange Value:
1 Fat Exchange + ½ Vegetable Exchange

TASTY STUFFED MUSHROOMS
(Serves 6)

½ pound whole fresh mushrooms
¼ cup grated Parmesan cheese
¼ cup bread crumbs
¼ teaspoon dried basil
¼ teaspoon dried oregano
⅛ teaspoon dried thyme

*W*ash the mushrooms and separate the stems from the caps. Combine the cheese, bread crumbs, basil, oregano, thyme, and mushroom stems in a food processor or blender and purée. Stuff the mixture into the mushroom caps. Bake in a 425-degree oven for about 5 minutes, or until the mushrooms are tender.

ONE SERVING
=
35 calories
3 CHO
2 PRO
2 FAT
90 SODIUM
33 POTASSIUM
3 CHOLESTEROL

Exchange Value:
1 Vegetable Exchange

PEARS WITH RICOTTA

(Serves 2)

2 small ripe pears
4 tablespoons ricotta cheese
1 tablespoon chopped pistachio nuts plus extra nuts
   for garnish

*C*ut the pears in half and remove the cores. Mix the
ricotta cheese with the nuts. Spread on the cut sides of
the pears. Garnish with the extra nuts.

**ONE
SERVING**
=
*152 calories
24 CHO
5 PRO
8 FAT
27 SODIUM
263 POTASSIUM
16 CHOLESTEROL*

*Exchange Value:
1½ Fruit Exchanges +
1 Lean Meat Exchange
+ 1 Fat Exchange*

CARROT–COTTAGE
CHEESE DIP

(Serves 6)

¾ cup lowfat cottage cheese
3 tablespoons plain lowfat yogurt
2 medium-size carrots, finely grated
¼ teaspoon ground white pepper
1 tablespoon caraway seeds
3 cups (total) broccoli flowerets, cucumber slices, green
   pepper strips, and cauliflower pieces

*C*ombine the cottage cheese, yogurt, carrots, pepper,
and caraway seeds in a bowl. Mix well or purée in a
blender or food processor. Cover and chill. Serve with
the vegetables.

**ONE
SERVING**
=
*40 calories
4 CHO
5 PRO
1 FAT
131 SODIUM
126 POTASSIUM
3 CHOLESTEROL*

*Exchange Value:
½ Lean Meat
Exchange + 1
Vegetable Exchange*

CHERRY TOMATOES
WITH CRAB

(Serves 12)

1 pint (12 medium size) tomatoes
¼ cup flaked crab meat
1 tablespoon plain lowfat yogurt
2 teaspoons finely chopped green onion (scallion) or
   shallot
¼ teaspoon dried tarragon
Pinch of cayenne pepper
2 teaspoons minced fresh parsley leaves

*C*ut off the top of each tomato. Scoop out the seeds with a small spoon. Refrigerate until ready to serve. Combine the remaining ingredients. Refrigerate until ready to serve. Drain off any juice in the tomatoes and crab mixture. Spoon the crab mixture into the tomatoes. Serve cold.

**ONE
SERVING**
=

11 calories
2 CHO
1 PRO
0 FAT
2 SODIUM
78 POTASSIUM
4 CHOLESTEROL

Exchange Value:
FREE

OYSTERS CASINO

(Serves 4—6 oysters per serving)

24 medium-size oysters
Lemon juice
¼ cup butter
2 tablespoons chopped green onion (scallion)
3 tablespoons chopped fresh parsley leaves
¼ cup minced celery

*A*rrange the oysters on the half shell in a baking pan. Sprinkle with lemon juice. Cream together the butter, onion, parsley, and celery. Spoon the butter mixture over the oysters. Bake in a 450-degree oven until the oysters curl at the edge.

ONE SERVING
=
228 calories
7 CHO
15 PRO
16 FAT
259 SODIUM
238 POTASSIUM
123 CHOLESTEROL

Exchange Value:
2 Lean Meat Exchanges + 2 Fat Exchanges + 1 Vegetable Exchange

MERRY CRANBERRY PUNCH

(Makes twenty 3-ounce servings)

2 cups (1 pint) cranberry juice cocktail
1 6-ounce can frozen grapefruit juice concentrate
3 cans water
1 teaspoon ground coriander
2 teaspoons grated orange peel
2 bottles champagne or dry white wine, well chilled
   (optional)
Thin orange slices

*C*ombine all the ingredients, *except* the champagne and orange slices. Chill until ready to serve. Just before serving, add the champagne and garnish with the orange slices.

ONE SERVING
=
66 calories
8 CHO
0 PRO
0 FAT
4 SODIUM
84 POTASSIUM
0 CHOLESTEROL

Exchange Value:
1 Fruit Exchange +
½ Fat Exchange

If made without the champagne or white wine:

ONE SERVING
=
25 calories
6 CHO
0 PRO
0 FAT
1 SODIUM
40 POTASSIUM
0 CHOLESTEROL

Exchange Value:
½ Fruit Exchange

RASPBERRY SMOOTHIE

(Serves 2)

¼ cup unsweetened pineapple juice
½ cup raspberries
3 ice cubes
1 large kiwi fruit, peeled and sliced

Combine all the ingredients in a blender and purée until smooth. Pour into champagne glasses. Serve garnished with a raspberry or kiwi slice.

ONE SERVING
=
56 calories
14 CHO
1 PRO
0 FAT
2 SODIUM
215 POTASSIUM
0 CHOLESTEROL

Exchange Value:
1 Fruit Exchange

KIWI–YOGURT SMOOTHIE

(Serves 2)

2 kiwi fruit, peeled and sliced
1 ripe banana, peeled
¼ cup plain lowfat yogurt
3 ice cubes
2 large strawberries

Combine the kiwi, banana, yogurt, and ice cubes in a blender. Purée until smooth. Pour into two glasses. Garnish each with a strawberry.

ONE SERVING
=
69 calories
22 CHO
2 PRO
1 FAT
25 SODIUM
653 POTASSIUM
2 CHOLESTEROL

Exchange Value:
1½ Fruit Exchanges

TOMATO COCKTAIL

(Serves 4)

3 cups diced peeled ripe tomatoes OR 2 cups canned
    tomato juice
3 green onions (scallions), cut into 2-inch pieces
¼ teaspoon salt (omit if canned juice is used)
1 teaspoon Worcestershire sauce
1 teaspooon dried basil
½ teaspoon celery seeds

Combine all the ingredients in a blender. Blend until
the mixture is completely liquefied. Chill until ready to
serve. Serve in chilled glasses garnished with a lemon
wedge, if desired.

ONE SERVING
=
41 calories
8 CHO
1 PRO
0 FAT
240 SODIUM
407 POTASSIUM
0 CHOLESTEROL

Exchange Value:
1 Vegetable Exchange

CRANBERRY COOLER

(Serves 6)

4 cups (1 quart) cranberry juice cocktail
1½ cups club soda

Combine the cranberry juice cocktail and club soda.
Pour over ice.

Note: To make 1 serving, mix ¾ cup cranberry juice
with ¼ cup club soda. Serve over ice.

ONE SERVING
=
58 calories
12 CHO
0 PRO
0 FAT
7 SODIUM
41 POTASSIUM
0 CHOLESTEROL

Exchange Value:
1 Fruit Exchange

FRUIT PUNCH

(Serves 12—½ cup per serving)

2 cups unsweetened pineapple juice, chilled
2 cups cranberry juice cocktail, chilled
¾ cup orange juice, chilled
¾ cup club soda, chilled
Ice cubes
Lime slices

Combine the chilled ingredients in a punch bowl just before serving.

**ONE
SERVING**
=
30 calories
7 CHO
0 PRO
0 FAT
0 SODIUM
85 POTASSIUM
0 CHOLESTEROL

Exchange Value:
1 Fruit Exchange

SPICY TOMATO COCKTAIL

(Serves 8—1 cup per serving)

1 cucumber
6 cups canned tomato juice
3 green onions (scallions), chopped
2 tablespoons lemon juice
Dash of Tabasco sauce
1 teaspoon Worcestershire sauce
1 tablespoon prepared horseradish

Peel and grate the cucumber. Add it to the tomato juice with the remaining ingredients. Cover and refrigerate for 2 hours or overnight. Strain before serving.

**ONE
SERVING**
=
38 calories
9 CHO
2 PRO
0 FAT
369 SODIUM
447 POTASSIUM
0 CHOLESTEROL

Exchange Value:
*2 Vegetable
Exchanges*

LOW-CALORIE EGGNOG

(Serves 8—½ cup per serving)

2 eggs, separated
4 cups skim milk
1 teaspoon vanilla extract
3 packets Equal sweetener
½ teaspoon brandy or rum flavoring
Ground nutmeg

Combine the egg yolks and milk in a saucepan. Cook over medium heat until the mixture coats a metal spoon. Cool.

Beat the egg whites until soft peaks form. Add to the egg custard mixture with the vanilla, sweetener, and flavoring. Mix lightly. Cover and chill. Pour into serving cups and sprinkle with nutmeg.

ONE SERVING
=
70 calories
6 CHO
6 PRO
3 FAT
80 SODIUM
207 POTASSIUM
74 CHOLESTEROL

Exchange Value:
½ Medium-Fat Meat
Exchange + ½ Milk
Exchange

HOT WASSAIL

(Serves 18—½ cup per serving)

4 cups (1 quart) unsweetened apple juice
3 cups unsweetened pineapple juice
2 cups cranberry juice cocktail
¼ teaspoon ground nutmeg
1 cinnamon stick
3 whole cloves
Lemon slices

Combine all the ingredients in a large kettle and simmer for 10 minutes. Serve hot.

ONE SERVING
=
65 calories
16 CHO
0 PRO
0 FAT
3 SODIUM
128 POTASSIUM
0 CHOLESTEROL

Exchange Value:
1 Fruit Exchange

CHRISTMAS CRANBERRY PUNCH

(Serves 16—¹/₂ cup per serving)

4 cups cranberry juice cocktail
2 cups orange juice
12 ounces sugar-free lemon-lime carbonated beverage
Whole cranberries
Holly leaves

Combine the cranberry and orange juices in a punch bowl. Pour the carbonated beverage down the sides of the bowl. Float whole cranberries and holly leaves on top.

**ONE
SERVING**
=
51 calories
13 CHO
0 PRO
0 FAT
3 SODIUM
75 POTASSIUM
0 CHOLESTEROL

Exchange Value:
1 Fruit Exchange

5

YUMMY SALADS
AND SOUPS

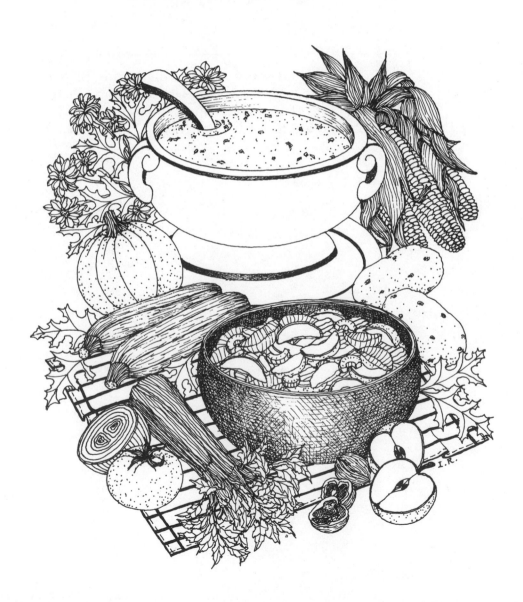

Salads and soups traditionally begin a meal. They can also be the main part of a lighter meal following that afternoon holiday feast.

TRADITIONAL WALDORF SALAD

(Serves 4)

2 large apples, cored and diced
2 teaspoons lemon juice
1 cup diced celery
2 tablespoons coarsely chopped walnuts
¼ cup dark or golden raisins
2 tablespoons mayonnaise or salad dressing
2 tablespoons lowfat milk
Lettuce leaves

*P*ut the apples in a medium-size bowl and add the lemon juice. Toss. Add the celery, walnuts, and raisins. In a small bowl, beat the mayonnaise and milk until smooth; toss with the apple mixture. Serve on lettuce.

ONE SERVING
=
147 calories
20 CHO
2 PRO
8 FAT
61 SODIUM
223 POTASSIUM
4 CHOLESTEROL

Exchange Value:
1½ Fruit Exchanges +
1½ Fat Exchanges

KIWI–TOMATO SALAD

(Serves 4)

Leaf or Bibb lettuce
4 kiwi fruit, peeled and sliced
2 celery stalks, chopped
2 ripe tomatoes, sliced
2 tablespoons vegetable oil
2 tablespoons lemon juice
2 tablespoons slivered almonds, toasted

*L*ine a salad bowl with the lettuce. Arrange the kiwi, celery, and tomato on the lettuce. Mix the oil and lemon juice together. Pour over the salad. Sprinkle on the almonds just before serving.

ONE SERVING
=
137 calories
15 CHO
2 PRO
9 FAT
22 SODIUM
464 POTASSIUM
0 CHOLESTEROL

Exchange Value:
1 Vegetable Exchange
+ ½ Fruit Exchange
+ 2 Fat Exchanges

FOUR-BEAN SALAD

(Serves 8)

1 10-ounce package frozen green beans
1 10-ounce package frozen lima beans
1 16-ounce can garbanzo beans (chick-peas), drained
1 16-ounce can red kidney beans, drained
1 sweet green pepper, sliced thin
1 sweet red onion, sliced thin
¾ cup French vinaigrette dressing
1 garlic clove, minced
1 tablespoon dried parsley flakes
½ teaspoon dried tarragon
½ teaspoon dried basil
Salad greens

Cook the green beans and lima beans until tender. Combine all the ingredients, *except* the salad greens, in a bowl. Toss lightly to mix. Cover and refrigerate for 2 to 3 hours or overnight. Serve on the salad greens.

ONE SERVING
=
219 calories
26 CHO
7 PRO
10 FAT
329 SODIUM
425 POTASSIUM
0 CHOLESTEROL

Exchange Value:
1 Bread Exchange +
2 Vegetable
Exchanges + 2 Fat
Exchanges

DIJON–BROCCOLI SALAD

(Serves 4)

3 cups broccoli flowerets and peeled stems
2 tablespoons vegetable oil
1 tablespoon red or white wine vinegar
1 garlic clove, minced
¼ cup orange juice
1 teaspoon Dijon mustard
¼ cup grated carrot

Steam the broccoli until it is just fork-tender. Combine the oil, vinegar, garlic, orange juice, and mustard and mix well. Add the broccoli to the dressing. Toss to combine. Serve warm or at room temperature. Sprinkle the carrot over the top before serving.

ONE SERVING
=
124 calories
8 CHO
4 PRO
10 FAT
35 SODIUM
444 POTASSIUM
0 CHOLESTEROL

Exchange Value:
1 Vegetable Exchange
+ 2 Fat Exchanges

LENTIL SALAD

(Serves 4)

1 cup dried lentils, sorted and washed
4 cups water
½ teaspoon salt
¼ cup chopped sweet green pepper
½ cup chopped onion
¼ cup chopped celery or cucumber
1 garlic clove, minced
1 tablespoon dried parsley flakes
¼ cup vegetable oil
2 tablespoons red or white wine vinegar
1 teaspoon salt
¼ teaspoon ground black pepper
¼ teaspoon ground cumin
2 hard-cooked eggs, cut into wedges

ONE SERVING
=
279 calories
23 CHO
12 PRO
17 FAT
757 SODIUM
755 POTASSIUM
137 CHOLESTEROL

Exchange Value:
1 Lean Meat
Exchange + 1 Bread
Exchange + 1
Vegetable Exchange
+ 3 Fat Exchanges

Cook the lentils in the water with ½ teaspoon of the salt until tender, about 20 minutes. Drain. Add the green pepper, onion, celery or cucumber, garlic, parsley, oil, vinegar, salt, pepper, and cumin. Toss lightly to mix. Cover and chill. Serve garnished with the egg wedges.

SLICED BEET SALAD

(Serves 2)

1½ cups sliced canned or cooked fresh beets
1 bay leaf
4 whole cloves
4 whole allspice
1 small grapefruit
1 package Equal sweetener

Drain the liquid from the canned beets, reserving ½ cup. (When using fresh beets, use water instead.) Combine the ½ cup beet liquid, bay leaf, cloves, and allspice in a small saucepan. Heat to boiling. Lower the heat and simmer for 5 minutes.

Section the grapefruit. Remove the spices from the liquid and pour over the beet slices and grapefruit sections. Add the sweetener. Marinate for at least 1 hour before serving. Drain off the liquid before serving.

ONE SERVING
=
86 calories
21 CHO
2 PRO
0 FAT
302 SODIUM
380 POTASSIUM
0 CHOLESTEROL

Exchange Value:
½ Fruit Exchange +
2 Vegetable
Exchanges

ZESTY ORANGE SALAD

(Serves 2)

2 oranges, peeled and sliced thin
1 small onion, sliced thin
2 teaspoons walnut or vegetable oil
1 tablespoon cider vinegar
⅛ teaspoon chili powder
Lettuce leaves

Combine all the ingredients, *except* the lettuce leaves, in a bowl. Cover and refrigerate for 2 hours before serving. Toss before serving on the lettuce leaves.

ONE SERVING
=
117 calories
19 CHO
2 PRO
5 FAT
4 SODIUM
301 POTASSIUM
0 CHOLESTEROL

Exchange Value:
1 Fruit Exchange +
1 Fat Exchange

HEARTS OF PALM SALAD
(Serves 4)

1 16-ounce can whole hearts of palm
1 small sweet green pepper, chopped
1 2-ounce jar sliced red pimientos, drained
1 celery stalk, chopped
2 green onions (scallions), sliced thin
1 tablespoon chopped fresh parsley leaves
2 tablespoons vegetable oil
¼ cup lemon juice
Lettuce leaves

ONE SERVING
=
90 calories
4 CHO
0 PRO
9 FAT
27 SODIUM
125 POTASSIUM
0 CHOLESTEROL

Exchange Value:
1 Vegetable Exchange
+ 2 Fat Exchanges

Drain the hearts of palm and cut them into bite-size pieces. Add the remaining ingredients, *except* the lettuce leaves, cover, and refrigerate overnight. Serve on lettuce leaves.

ORANGE WALDORF SALAD
(Serves 4)

4 oranges, peeled
1 apple
½ cup sliced celery
¼ cup plain lowfat yogurt
¼ cup chopped pecans, toasted
⅛ teaspoon ground cinnamon
Salad greens

ONE SERVING
=
145 calories
23 CHO
3 PRO
6 FAT
18 SODIUM
376 POTASSIUM
1 CHOLESTEROL

Exchange Value:
½ Vegetable Exchange + 1½ Fruit Exchanges + 1 Fat Exchange

Chop up orange and apple into bite-size pieces. Combine all the ingredients, *except* the salad greens, in a bowl. Cover and refrigerate. Serve on salad greens.

FRESH CAULIFLOWER SALAD

(Serves 2)

½ small head fresh cauliflower
1 tablespoon grated Parmesan cheese
½ tablespoon mayonnaise
¼ cup plain lowfat yogurt
Romaine or Bibb lettuce leaves
Minced fresh parsley leaves
Cherry tomatoes

*B*reak the cauliflower into small flowerets. Slice the stems into bite-size pieces. Combine the cauliflower, Parmesan cheese, mayonnaise, and yogurt in a bowl. Toss gently. Serve on lettuce and top with the minced parsley and cherry tomatoes.

**ONE
SERVING**
=
96 calories
8 CHO
6 PRO
6 FAT
109 SODIUM
367 POTASSIUM
7 CHOLESTEROL

*Exchange Value:
2 Vegetable
Exchanges + 1 Fat
Exchange*

CUCUMBER SALAD

(Serves 6)

1 large cucumber
2 large ripe tomatoes OR 1 pint cherry tomatoes
1 sweet green pepper
1 cup sliced carrots, steamed
¼ cup vegetable oil
¼ cup red or white wine vinegar
1 teaspoon ground coriander seeds
1 package Equal sweetener

*P*eel the cucumber; then cut in half lengthwise and remove the seeds. Cut the cucumber into thin slices. Peel the tomatoes and remove the seeds. Cut each into 8 wedges. (If cherry tomatoes are used, cut each in half.) Cut the green pepper in half. Remove the seeds and chop into ¼-inch pieces. Combine the cucumber, tomato, green pepper, and carrots in a bowl. Add the remaining ingredients and toss. Cover and refrigerate for at least 2 hours before serving.

ONE SERVING
=
110 calories
7 CHO
1 PRO
9 FAT
22 SODIUM
285 POTASSIUM
0 CHOLESTEROL

Exchange Value:
1 Vegetable Exchange
+ 2 Fat Exchanges

WILD RICE WALDORF SALAD

(Serves 4)

1 cup wild rice, cooked
1 apple, chopped
1 cup seedless grapes
1 cup chopped celery
2 tablespoons mayonnaise
1 tablespoon plain lowfat yogurt
2 tablespoons chopped dry roasted peanuts

*C*ombine all the ingredients, *except* the peanuts, in a bowl. Toss to mix. Cover and chill thoroughly, about 3 to 4 hours. Sprinkle the peanuts on top just before serving.

ONE SERVING
=
157 calories
20 CHO
3 PRO
7 FAT
138 SODIUM
193 POTASSIUM
4 CHOLESTEROL

Exchange Value:
1 Bread Exchange +
½ Fruit Exchange +
1 Fat Exchange

CRANBERRY RELISH

(Serves 6—½ cup per serving)

4 cups fresh or frozen cranberries
1 cup orange juice
8 packets Equal sweetener

*C*ook the cranberries with the orange juice until thick. Cool. Add the sweetener. Cover and refrigerate until ready to serve.

ONE SERVING
=
49 calories
12 CHO
0 PRO
0 FAT
1 SODIUM
124 POTASSIUM
0 CHOLESTEROL

Exchange Value:
1 Fruit Exchange

CRANAPPLE RELISH

(Serves 6—½ cup per serving)

1 apple
1 navel orange, peeled
2 cups fresh or frozen cranberries
½ teaspoon ground coriander
2 packets Equal sweetener

Shred the apple in a food processor or with a hand grater. Quarter the orange and combine with the cranberries in a food processor or food grinder. Process until coarsely chopped. Blend the apples, cranberry mixture, coriander, and sweetener together. Cover and refrigerate until ready to serve.

ONE SERVING
=
39 calories
10 CHO
0 PRO
0 FAT
0 SODIUM
88 POTASSIUM
0 CHOLESTEROL

Exchange Value:
½ Fruit Exchange

FRENCH DRESSING

(Serves 12)

½ teaspoon powdered mustard
¼ teaspoon ground white pepper
1 teaspoon tomato paste
7 tablespoons salad oil
⅓ cup red or white wine vinegar
2 teaspoons water
½ teaspoon finely chopped onion

Combine all the ingredients in a jar and shake well before using. For a smooth dressing, purée in a blender or food processor.

ONE TABLESPOON
=
50 calories
0 CHO
0 PRO
6 FAT
0 SODIUM
1 POTASSIUM
0 CHOLESTEROL

Exchange Value:
1 Fat Exchange

FRESH ITALIAN DRESSING

(Makes 1½ cups)

1 teaspoon chopped fresh thyme leaves
1 teaspoon chopped fresh basil leaves
2 teaspoons chopped fresh tarragon leaves
½ teaspoon ground white pepper
1 tablespoon minced onion
1 garlic clove
½ cup water
⅓ cup red or white wine vinegar
½ cup vegetable oil

Combine all the ingredients in a blender. Purée until smooth. For best flavor, make the dressing at least 3 hours before using.

Note: If fresh herbs are not available, use one-half the amounts of dried herbs.

ONE TABLESPOON
=
47 calories
0 CHO
0 PRO
5 FAT
0 SODIUM
5 POTASSIUM
0 CHOLESTEROL

Exchange Value:
1 Fat Exchange

DIJON MUSTARD DRESSING

(Makes ½ cup)

¼ cup red wine vinegar
½ teaspoon Dijon mustard
1 small garlic clove
1 tablespoon minced fresh parsley leaves OR 2 teaspoons dried parsley flakes
¼ cup vegetable oil

Combine all the ingredients in a food processor or blender. Process until smooth. Cover and refrigerate until ready to serve.

ONE TABLESPOON
=
62 calories
0 CHO
0 PRO
7 FAT
4 SODIUM
8 POTASSIUM
0 CHOLESTEROL

Exchange Value:
1 Fat Exchange

CREAMY GARLIC DRESSING

(Makes 1 cup)

1 cup lowfat cottage cheese
2 garlic cloves
¼ teaspoon ground white pepper
¼ cup skim milk
2 teaspoons prepared mustard
2 teaspoons lemon juice

*B*lend all the ingredients together in a food processor or blender until smooth. Chill for at least 3 hours before serving.

TWO TABLESPOONS
=
32 calories
1 CHO
4 PRO
1 FAT
110 SODIUM
38 POTASSIUM
4 CHOLESTEROL

Exchange Value:
½ Lean Meat
Exchange

PURÉE OF BROCCOLI SOUP

(Serves 10—½ cup per serving)

4 cups chicken broth
2 pounds fresh or frozen broccoli, chopped
1 medium-size potato, peeled and cubed
3 green onions (scallions), sliced thin
¼ teaspoon ground black pepper
2 tablespoons dried parsley flakes
½ teaspoon salt
1 bay leaf
½ teaspoon dried thyme

*C*ombine all the ingredients in large saucepan or slow cooker. Simmer until the broccoli is tender. Purée in food processor or blender. Heat if necessary before serving.

ONE SERVING
=
38 calories
8 CHO
2 PRO
0 FAT
105 SODIUM
264 POTASSIUM
0 CHOLESTEROL

Exchange Value:
1½ Vegetable
Exchanges

VEGETABLE–BARLEY SOUP

(Serves 15—1 cup per serving)

4 carrots, sliced
4 celery stalks, sliced
1 onion, chopped
1 rutabaga, peeled and cubed
2 parsnips, peeled and sliced
½ cup chopped fresh parsley leaves
2 cups sliced mushrooms
4 quarts (16 cups) water
1 28-ounce can crushed tomatoes
½ cup pearl barley

ONE SERVING
=
51 calories
10 CHO
2 PRO
0 FAT
72 SODIUM
252 POTASSIUM
0 CHOLESTEROL

Exchange Value:
2 Vegetable
Exchanges

Combine all the ingredients in a large saucepan.
Cover and cook for approximately 1 hour.

SAVORY POTATO SOUP

(Serves 6—½ cup per serving)

3 cups diced peeled potatoes
1 cup chopped celery
½ cup chopped onion
1 teaspoon salt
Pinch of ground white pepper
3 cups skim milk
2 tablespoons flour
2 tablespoons margarine
1 teaspoon dried dill

ONE SERVING
=
172 calories
26 CHO
7 PRO
3 FAT
448 SODIUM
636 POTASSIUM
5 CHOLESTEROL

Exchange Value:
1 Bread Exchange +
½ Milk Exchange +
1 Vegetable Exchange

Cook the potatoes, celery, onion, salt, and pepper in
just enough water to cover until the potatoes are
tender.

Meanwhile, combine the flour, margarine, and dill in
a skillet. Add the milk gradually and blend to make a
smooth sauce. Cook for 5 minutes. Add the potato
mixture and heat thoroughly.

CABBAGE SOUP

(Serves 6—½ cup per serving)

4 cups water
3 cups shredded cabbage
1 small onion, sliced
1 15-ounce can tomato sauce OR 5 ripe tomatoes
2 tablespoons dark or golden raisins
1 teaspoon caraway seeds
½ teaspoon salt

Combine all the ingredients in a slow cooker or large saucepan. Cook for 2 to 3 hours in the slow cooker or 1 hour over medium heat.

ONE SERVING
=
32 calories
7 CHO
1 PRO
0 FAT
224 SODIUM
215 POTASSIUM
0 CHOLESTEROL

Exchange Value:
1 Vegetable Exchange

LOW-CALORIE MINESTRONE

(Serves 12—1 cup per serving)

8 cups chicken or turkey broth
1½ cups chopped celery
1 cup chopped onion
1 medium-size zucchini, sliced
2 16-ounce cans tomatoes OR 10 ripe tomatoes, peeled
2 cups finely chopped cabbage
¼ cup chopped fresh parsley leaves
1 garlic clove, minced
1 bay leaf
1 teaspoon dried thyme
½ teaspoon salt
½ teaspoon ground black pepper

Combine all the ingredients in a saucepan. Simmer for 30 minutes, or until the vegetables are tender.

ONE SERVING
=
35 calories
8 CHO
2 PRO
0 FAT
97 SODIUM
346 POTASSIUM
0 CHOLESTEROL

Exchange Value:
1 Vegetable Exchange

TOMATO–SHRIMP CHOWDER

(Serves 8—½ cup per serving)

2 cups canned tomato juice
2 cups peeled and chopped tomatoes
1 cup chopped celery
½ cup sliced onion
½ cup sliced carrots
1 teaspoon dried parsley flakes
4 whole cloves
6 whole black peppercorns
1 small bay leaf
⅛ teaspoon dried thyme
¼ cup brown rice
1 pound medium-size shrimp, shelled and deveined
Thin lemon slices

ONE SERVING
=
96 calories
13 CHO
10 PRO
1 FAT
176 SODIUM
510 POTASSIUM
68 CHOLESTEROL

Exchange Value:
2 Lean Meat
Exchanges + 2
Vegetable Exchanges

Combine all the ingredients, *except* the shrimp and lemon slices, in a large saucepan. Bring to a boil, lower the heat, and simmer for 40 to 50 minutes. Purée in a blender until smooth. Steam the shrimp and add them to the tomato mixture. Garnish with the lemon slices just before serving.

ACORN SQUASH SOUP

(Serves 6—½ cup per serving)

2 small acorn squash
1 leek or small onion, chopped fine (Wash the leek
  well.)
1 tablespoon vegetable oil
1 carrot, sliced thin
3 cups chicken or turkey broth
1 apple, peeled, cored, and diced
1 bay leaf
¼ teaspoon curry powder
½ teaspoon dried parsley flakes
Pinch of ground cinnamon
6 teaspoons grated Parmesan cheese

*C*ut the squash into quarters and remove the seeds.
Steam the squash until soft. Sauté the leek in the oil.
Add the carrot, chicken or turkey broth, apple, bay
leaf, curry powder, and parsley. Scoop out the pulp
from the squash and add it to the mixture. Cook over
medium heat until the carrots are soft. Remove the bay
leaf. Mash with a potato masher or purée in a blender
or food processor. Pour into serving bowls and
sprinkle with cinnamon and one teaspoon of cheese
per serving. Reheat if necessary before serving.

ONE SERVING

=

128 calories
16 CHO
2 PRO
7 FAT
39 SODIUM
398 POTASSIUM
1 CHOLESTEROL

Exchange Value:
1 Bread Exchange +
1 Fat Exchange

ONION SOUP

(Serves 5—1 cup per serving)

5 cups water
Beef soup bones (fat trimmed) OR 4 ounces lean beef,
   cut into cubes
2 large onions
2 teaspoons vegetable oil
15 whole black peppercorns OR ¼ teaspoon ground
   black pepper
2 bay leaves
¼ teaspoon dried thyme
½ teaspoon salt (optional)
Grated Parmesan cheese

Combine the water and soup bones or beef in a
saucepan. Cook for 4 hours or overnight in a slow
cooker. Remove the soup bones or beef. Slice the
onions and sauté in a skillet in the vegetable oil until
brown and tender. Add to the beef stock along with
the peppercorns (or pepper), bay leaves, thyme, and
salt (optional). Simmer for 30 minutes to 1 hour to
blend the flavors. Remove the peppercorns and bay
leaves before serving. Serve with a teaspoon of grated
cheese on top.

**ONE
SERVING**
=

*85 calories
3 CHO
7 PRO
5 FAT
55 SODIUM
118 POTASSIUM
22 CHOLESTEROL*

*Exchange Value:
1 Medium-Fat Meat
Exchange*

CHICKEN–RICE SOUP

(Serves 6—1 cup per serving)

1 3-pound chicken, cut into pieces
8 cups water
½ cup chopped celery with leaves
¼ cup chopped fresh parsley leaves
1 small onion
½ teaspoon whole white peppercorns
1 bay leaf
¼ teaspoon celery seeds
½ cup rice, uncooked
1 cup diced carrots

Simmer the chicken in the water with the celery, parsley, onion, peppercorns, bay leaf, and celery seeds for 4 hours in a slow cooker or 1 hour over low heat on the range. Drain the chicken broth and remove the chicken pieces. Bone the chicken and chop it into bite-size pieces. Combine the broth, chicken, rice, and carrots in a saucepan. Cook for 30 to 40 minutes, or until the rice is tender.

ONE SERVING
=

287 calories
11 CHO
29 PRO
10 FAT
219 SODIUM
307 POTASSIUM
88 CHOLESTEROL

Exchange Value:
3 Lean Meat
Exchanges + ½
Bread Exchange

HEARTY LENTIL SOUP

(Serves 6—½ cup per serving)

2 cups dried lentils, sorted and washed
1 garlic clove, finely chopped
1 medium-size onion, sliced
2 large carrots, sliced
1 large celery stalk, sliced
4 cups water
1 teaspoon soy sauce (optional)
2 tablespoons chopped fresh parsley leaves
1 teaspoon salt
½ teaspoon ground black pepper
1 bay leaf
¼ teaspoon dried thyme
1 28-ounce can whole tomatoes

**ONE
SERVING**
=
*105 calories
20 CHO
7 PRO
0 FAT
449 SODIUM
468 POTASSIUM
0 CHOLESTEROL*

*Exchange Value:
1 Lean Meat
Exchange + 1 Bread
Exchange*

Cover the lentils with water in a large saucepan and bring to a boil. Boil, uncovered, for 2 minutes. Remove from the heat, cover, and let stand for 1 hour. Add the remaining ingredients, *except* the tomatoes. Heat to boiling. Lower the heat, cover, and simmer for 1 hour. Stir in the tomatoes and liquid. Simmer, uncovered, for 15 minutes.

GREEN SPLIT PEA SOUP

(Serves 6—½ cup per serving)

3 cups water
½ cup brown rice, uncooked
1 cup split peas
½ teaspoon salt
⅓ cup chopped onion
1 tablespoon vegetable oil
½ cup diced carrots
½ cup diced celery
½ teaspoon dried basil

*B*ring the water to a boil and add the rice. Cover and cook for 30 minutes. Stir in the peas and cook over medium heat for 30 minutes. Sauté the onion in the vegetable oil. Add the salt, onion, carrots, and celery. Cook for 15 minutes, or just until the vegetables are tender. Sprinkle with the basil.

ONE SERVING
=
82 calories
13 CHO
3 PRO
3 FAT
220 SODIUM
164 POTASSIUM
0 CHOLESTEROL

Exchange Value:
1 Bread Exchange +
½ Fat Exchange

OYSTER STEW

(Serves 4—½ cup per serving)

1 pint oysters and oyster liquor
1 tablespoon butter
2 cups lowfat milk
⅛ teaspoon cayenne pepper
Chopped fresh parsley leaves

*C*ombine the oysters, oyster liquor, and butter in a skillet. Cook until the edges of the oysters curl. Add the milk. Heat just to boiling. Sprinkle with the pepper. Ladle into hot bowls. Garnish with the parsley.

ONE SERVING
=
154 calories
10 CHO
14 PRO
7 FAT
184 SODIUM
337 POTASSIUM
65 CHOLESTEROL

Exchange Value:
1 Lean Meat
Exchange + 1 Milk
Exchange + 1 Fat
Exchange

6

VEGETABLES AND FRUITS TO ADD MENU GLAMOUR

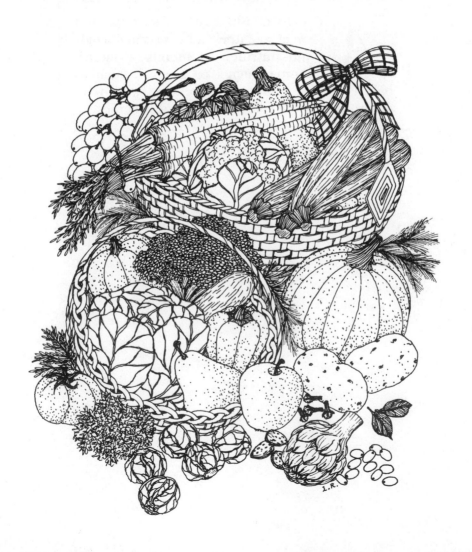

Acorn squash, Brussels sprouts, and sweet potatoes add seasonal color and nutrition to menus. Fruit accompaniments to a meal, such as baked apples, cranberry toppings, and fruit ambrosia provide color and natural sweetness.

RATATOUILLE

(Serves 4)

1 small sweet green pepper
1 medium-size onion
1 teaspoon vegetable oil
1 medium-size ripe tomato
1 medium-size zucchini (½ pound)
1 small eggplant (¾ pound)
1 garlic clove, minced
½ teaspoon dried basil
½ teaspoon dried thyme
2 tablespoons minced fresh parsley leaves

*C*ut the green pepper into strips. Slice the onion. Sauté the pepper and onion in the oil. Chop the tomato and slice the zucchini into ¼-inch-thick slices. Cube the eggplant. Add the tomato, zucchini, eggplant, garlic, basil, thyme, and parsley to the pepper and onion mixture. Simmer until the vegetables are tender.

ONE SERVING

=

47 calories
8 CHO
2 PRO
2 FAT
7 SODIUM
306 POTASSIUM
0 CHOLESTEROL

Exchange Value:
2 Vegetable Exchanges

ZUCCHINI MANDARIN

(Serves 4)

1 pound zucchini
1 8-ounce can mandarin oranges, drained
¼ teaspoon ground nutmeg
¼ cup slivered almonds, toasted

*C*ut the zucchini into slices. Steam until tender. Add the orange slices and nutmeg. Sprinkle with the almonds just before serving.

ONE SERVING

=

60 calories
8 CHO
2 PRO
3 FAT
1 SODIUM
239 POTASSIUM
0 CHOLESTEROL

Exchange Value:
½ Fruit Exchange +
½ Fat Exchange

ITALIAN STEAMED ARTICHOKES

(Serves 1)

1 large artichoke (about 1 pound)
1 garlic clove, sliced thin
1 bay leaf
¼ teaspoon coriander seeds
½ teaspoon dried oregano
½ teaspoon dried basil

Snip the thorns off the artichoke leaves. Place the garlic slices inside the leaves throughout the artichoke. Put the artichoke into a medium-size saucepan. Add water to come halfway up the artichoke. Put the bay leaf in the water. Crush the coriander seeds, oregano, and basil together. Sprinkle on top of the artichoke. Cook over medium heat for 30 minutes, or until the leaves pull off easily.

**ONE
SERVING**
=

44 calories
10 CHO
3 PRO
0 FAT
30 SODIUM
301 POTASSIUM
0 CHOLESTEROL

Exchange Value:
2 Vegetable
Exchanges

FENNEL AND RICE
(Serves 4)

1 medium-size fennel bulb
1 sweet red pepper
1 small onion, chopped
1 tablespoon vegetable oil
½ cup brown rice
1 bay leaf
2 cups water

*T*rim off the top of the fennel bulb. Cut the fennel into small cubes. Clean the pepper and cut it into small cubes. Combine the fennel, pepper, onion, and vegetable oil in a saucepan. Cook over medium heat for 2 minutes. Add the rice, bay leaf, and water. Bring to a boil, cover, and turn the heat to low. Cook for 30 to 35 minutes, or until the rice is tender.

ONE SERVING
=
103 calories
16 CHO
2 PRO
4 FAT
159 SODIUM
162 POTASSIUM
0 CHOLESTEROL

Exchange Value:
1 Bread Exchange +
1 Fat Exchange

VEGETABLE CONFETTI
(Serves 2)

1 small zucchini, shredded
1 small yellow squash, shredded
2 carrots, shredded
1 small onion, sliced thin
2 tablespoons water
2 teaspoons margarine

*C*ombine the zucchini, yellow squash, carrots, onion, and water in a skillet. Cover and cook over medium heat for 4 to 5 minutes, or until the vegetables are tender. Add the margarine. Sauté, uncovered, until all the moisture has evaporated. Serve immediately.

ONE SERVING
=
94 calories
14 CHO
3 PRO
4 FAT
83 SODIUM
453 POTASSIUM
0 CHOLESTEROL

Exchange Value:
2 Vegetable
Exchanges + 1 Fat
Exchange

BUTTERNUT SQUASH WITH GINGER

(Serves 4)

1 large butternut squash
1 tablespoon minced fresh gingerroot
¼ cup unsweetened apple juice
Freshly ground nutmeg

*P*eel and seed the squash. Cut it into ½-inch cubes. Put the squash, gingerroot, and apple juice into a lightly oiled baking dish. Cover and bake in a 350-degree oven for 50 to 60 minutes. Sprinkle on the nutmeg just before serving.

ONE SERVING
=
70 calories
17 CHO
2 PRO
0 FAT
2 SODIUM
480 POTASSIUM
0 CHOLESTEROL

Exchange Value:
1 Bread Exchange

WILD RICE-STUFFED SQUASH

(Serves 4)

2 medium-size acorn squash
½ cup wild rice, cooked
1 teaspoon grated orange rind
½ cup chopped walnuts
1 to 2 tablespoons frozen orange juice concentrate

*C*ut the squash in half and remove the seeds. Combine the remaining ingredients and fill the squash with the mixture. Place in a baking pan. Cover with aluminum foil or a lid and bake in a 400-degree oven for about 35 minutes, or until the squash is fork-tender. Extra orange juice concentrate can be drizzled over the squash just before serving.

ONE SERVING
=
204 calories
28 CHO
5 PRO
10 FAT
20 SODIUM
610 POTASSIUM
0 CHOLESTEROL

Exchange Value:
2 Bread Exchanges
+ 2 Fat Exchanges

CRANBERRY-STUFFED ACORN SQUASH

(Serves 4)

2 medium-size acorn squash
1 apple, chopped
½ cup chopped fresh or frozen cranberries
1 orange, peeled and chopped
½ teaspoon ground cinnamon
2 teaspoons honey or Equal sweetener

*C*ut the squash in half and remove the seeds.
Combine the remaining ingredients, *except* the honey
or sweetener. Fill the squash with the mixture. Drizzle
the honey or sweetener over the squash. Place in a
baking pan. Cover with aluminum foil or a lid and
bake for 25 minutes in a 400-degree oven. Remove the
foil and continue baking until the squash is tender,
about 20 minutes.

ONE SERVING
=
125 calories
31 CHO
2 PRO
1 FAT
2 SODIUM
608 POTASSIUM
0 CHOLESTEROL

Exchange Value:
1 Bread Exchange +
1½ Fruit Exchanges

BAKED ZUCCHINI WITH CHEESE

(Serves 3)

2 medium-size zucchini, sliced very thin
1 egg
1 teaspoon prepared mustard
⅛ teaspoon ground white pepper
⅛ teaspoon ground nutmeg
1 green onion (scallion), sliced thin
½ cup grated lowfat Swiss cheese

*P*ut the zucchini in a colander or on towels to drain off the moisture. Combine the remaining ingredients. Add the zucchini and mix well. Pour into a lightly oiled 2-quart casserole. Bake in a 350-degree oven for 40 to 45 minutes.

ONE SERVING
=
72 calories
3 CHO
5 PRO
5 FAT
69 SODIUM
128 POTASSIUM
100 CHOLESTEROL

Exchange Value:
½ Medium-Fat Meat Exchange + 1 Vegetable Exchange

BRUSSELS SPROUTS WITH WALNUTS

(Serves 4)

2 cups fresh Brussels sprouts
¼ cup chopped walnuts
1 tablespoon margarine
¼ teaspoon ground nutmeg

*C*ut the Brussels sprouts in half and steam them until they are tender.

Meanwhile, sauté the walnuts in the margarine until golden. Pour over the sprouts in a serving dish. Sprinkle on the nutmeg.

ONE SERVING
=
100 calories
6 CHO
4 PRO
8 FAT
44 SODIUM
27 POTASSIUM
0 CHOLESTEROL

Exchange Value:
1 Vegetable Exchange + 1½ Fat Exchanges

BAKED STUFFED PUMPKIN

(Serves 8)

1 2-pound pumpkin
2 apples, cored and quartered
½ cup pineapple chunks
½ cup broken walnuts
1 teaspoon ground cinnamon
½ teaspoon ground nutmeg
¼ teaspoon ground cloves

*C*ut the top off the pumpkin and remove the seeds from the pumpkin. Place cut side down in a baking pan and bake in a 350-degree oven for about 40 minutes, or until soft.

　With a metal spoon, scrape out the cooked pumpkin, leaving a ⅛- to ¼-inch thick shell. Process the apples in a food processor until chunky. Add the remaining ingredients and process just until mixed. Spoon into the pumpkin shell. Cover with the top. Bake in a 400-degree oven for 45 minutes, or until the filling is hot.

ONE SERVING
=
118 calories
18 CHO
3 PRO
5 FAT
3 SODIUM
376 POTASSIUM
0 CHOLESTEROL

Exchange Value:
1 Vegetable Exchange
+ 1 Fruit Exchange
+ 1 Fat Exchange

CAULIFLOWER PIQUANTE

(Serves 6)

4 cups fresh cauliflower pieces
⅓ cup vegetable oil
2 tablespoons cider vinegar
½ teaspoon dried dill
Pinch of ground white pepper

*S*team the cauliflower until it is just crisp-tender. Combine with the remaining ingredients in a bowl. Stir to coat. Let stand at room temperature for 1 hour before serving. If made in advance, refrigerate after marinating for 1 hour.

ONE SERVING
=
125 calories
4 CHO
2 PRO
12 FAT
9 SODIUM
197 POTASSIUM
0 CHOLESTEROL

Exchange Value:
1 Vegetable Exchange
+ 2 Fat Exchanges

OVEN-BAKED HERB POTATOES

(Serves 4)

2 medium-size baking potatoes
1 tablespoon vegetable oil
½ teaspoon dried thyme
½ teaspoon dried oregano

Slice the potatoes about ¼ inch thick. Brush the slices with the vegetable oil. Place in a baking pan. Sprinkle with the thyme and oregano. Bake in a 400-degree oven for 15 to 20 minutes, or until tender.

ONE SERVING
=
102 calories
17 CHO
2 PRO
4 FAT
3 SODIUM
396 POTASSIUM
0 CHOLESTEROL

Exchange Value:
1 Bread Exchange +
1 Fat Exchange

CRANBERRY–RAISIN SAUCE

(Serves 4)

1 cup orange juice
½ cup fresh or frozen cranberries
1 tablespoon cornstarch
⅛ teaspoon ground cloves
4 tablespoons dark or golden raisins
Cinnamon stick

Combine the juice and cranberries in a saucepan. Cook over medium heat just until the berries "pop." Add the remaining ingredients and cook until the mixture is thick. Serve hot over baked ham.

ONE SERVING OF ¼ CUP
=
41 calories
10 CHO
1 PRO
0 FAT
0 SODIUM
127 POTASSIUM
0 CHOLESTEROL

Exchange Value:
1 Fruit Exchange

CRANBERRY SWEET POTATOES

(Serves 6)

6 sweet potatoes
½ cup frozen orange juice concentrate
2 cups fresh or frozen cranberries
Equal sweetener to taste (optional)

*B*ake the sweet potatoes in a 400-degree oven for about 40 minutes, or until they are soft. Combine the orange juice concentrate and cranberries in a saucepan. Bring to a boil. Lower the heat and simmer until the cranberries pop and the sauce thickens. Add the sweetener, if desired. Cut the tops of the sweet potatoes open and press open from the bottom. Top each potato with the cranberry orange sauce.

ONE SERVING
=
213 calories
40 CHO
4 PRO
1 FAT
12 SODIUM
522 POTASSIUM
0 CHOLESTEROL

Exchange Value:
1 Bread Exchange +
2 Fruit Exchanges

BAKED APPLES WITH RAISINS

(Serves 2)

2 apples
Orange juice
1 tablespoon dark or golden raisins
Pinch of ground cinnamon

*P*eel and core the apples. Coat with the orange juice on the outer surface. Stuff with the raisins. Sprinkle on the cinnamon. Place in Pyrex baking cups. Bake in a 350-degree oven for 25 to 30 minutes, or until fork pierces surface easily. Serve warm or cold.

ONE SERVING
=
74 calories
19 CHO
0 PRO
0 FAT
0 SODIUM
105 POTASSIUM
0 CHOLESTEROL

Exchange Value:
1½ Fruit Exchanges

SWEET POTATOES
À L'ORANGE

(Serves 4)

2 pounds sweet potatoes, cooked, OR 2 pounds
   vacuum-packed sweet potatoes
2 tablespoons margarine, melted
½ teaspoon ground cinnamon
16 dried apricot halves
Fresh orange slices

*A*rrange the sweet potatoes in a shallow baking dish.
Combine the margarine and cinnamon. Pour over the
potatoes. Arrange the apricot halves on top. Cover the
dish and bake in a 425-degree oven for about 15
minutes. Add the orange slices and serve.

**ONE
SERVING**
=
*185 calories
23 CHO
3 PRO
7 FAT
79 SODIUM
526 POTASSIUM
0 CHOLESTEROL*

*Exchange Value:
1 Bread Exchange +
1 Fruit Exchange +
1 Fat Exchange*

PICKLED BEETS

(Serves 4)

1 cup sliced cooked beets
1 bay leaf, crumbled
¼ teaspoon whole black peppercorns
¼ cup sliced onion
¼ cup cider vinegar

*C*ombine all the ingredients in a saucepan. Bring to a
boil and remove from the heat. Serve hot or cold.

**ONE
SERVING**
=
*22 calories
6 CHO
1 PRO
0 FAT
102 SODIUM
102 POTASSIUM
0 CHOLESTEROL*

*Exchange Value:
1 Vegetable Exchange*

FRESH FRUIT AMBROSIA

(Serves 6—1/2 cup per serving)

¼ cup orange juice
½ cup club soda
1 medium-size banana, peeled
3 cups fresh fruit pieces (such as cantaloupe, grapes,
    pineapple, apple, pear, nectarine, plum, honeydew
    melon, blueberries, strawberries)
½ teaspoon ground nutmeg
¼ teaspoon ground cardamom
1 tablespoon sweetened coconut (flaked or shredded),
    toasted

ONE SERVING
=

81 calories
20 CHO
1 PRO
1 FAT
1 SODIUM
278 POTASSIUM
0 CHOLESTEROL

Exchange Value:
1½ Fruit Exchanges

Combine the orange juice, club soda, and banana in a blender and purée until smooth. Pour over the fresh fruit mixture. Sprinkle with the nutmeg and cardamom. Cover and refrigerate until ready to serve. Sprinkle on the coconut and serve immediately.

7

Stuffings, Dressings, and Casseroles

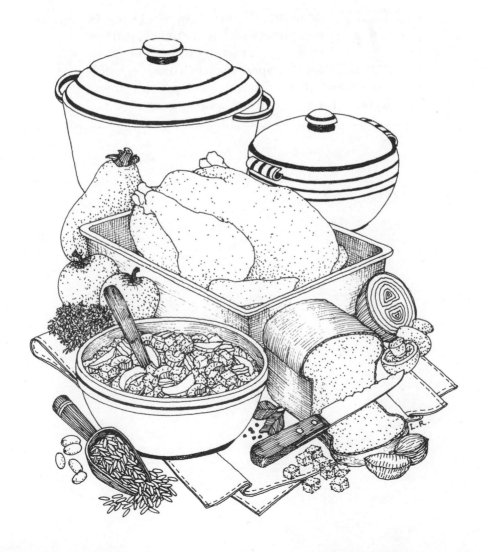

For many, the holidays would not be complete without a turkey stuffing or a corn bread dressing. The casserole recipes that feature vegetable proteins and dairy products will provide menu selections for a vegetarian holiday guest.

LOW-CALORIE APPLE DRESSING

(Serves 2)

1 apple, chopped
1 celery stalk, chopped
1 green onion (scallion), minced
½ teaspoon ground sage
¼ teaspoon dried thyme

*C*ombine all the ingredients in a bowl and toss. Spoon into a small baking dish. Cover with aluminum foil and bake in a 325-degree oven for about 30 minutes. Or use to stuff a Cornish hen. Double the recipe to use as a stuffing for a chicken.

ONE SERVING
=
58 calories
15 CHO
1 PRO
0 FAT
15 SODIUM
172 POTASSIUM
0 CHOLESTEROL

Exchange Value:
1 Fruit Exchange +
1 Vegetable Exchange

CORN BREAD STUFFING

(Serves 8)

1 recipe corn bread, crumbled (see recipe page 143)
1 cup chopped celery
1 small onion, chopped
1 egg
½ teaspoon dried sage
½ teaspoon ground black pepper
1 teaspoon dried thyme
1 tablespoon dried parsley flakes
½ teaspoon celery seeds
½ cup chicken or turkey broth or water

*C*ombine all the ingredients in a mixing bowl. Stuff into an 8- to 10-pound turkey. Or use to stuff two 3-pound chickens.

ONE SERVING
=
149 calories
22 CHO
4 PRO
5 FAT
215 SODIUM
91 POTASSIUM
58 CHOLESTEROL

Exchange Value:
1 Bread Exchange +
1 Vegetable Exchange
+ 1 Fat Exchange

PECAN CORN BREAD STUFFING

(Serves 8)

2 cups corn bread crumbs (see recipe page 143)
½ cup finely chopped onion
¼ cup chopped pecans
½ cup chopped celery
1 tablespoon dried parsley flakes
½ teaspoon dried thyme
¼ cup water or chicken broth

Mix all the ingredients together in a bowl. Stuff into poultry or transfer to a lightly oiled casserole. Bake in a 350-degree oven for 15 minutes if not used as a stuffing. Use as stuffing for two Cornish hens or one 3-pound chicken.

ONE SERVING
=

168 calories
22 CHO
3 PRO
6 FAT
202 SODIUM
110 POTASSIUM
23 CHOLESTEROL

Exchange Value:
1 Bread Exchange +
1 Vegetable Exchange
+ 1 Fat Exchange

BREAD STUFFING

(Serves 4)

4 cups dry bread cubes
1 cup chopped celery
1 onion, chopped
2 tablespoons chopped fresh parsley leaves
1 garlic clove, minced
1 cup hot water or turkey broth
¼ teaspoon ground black pepper
¾ teaspoon ground sage
¼ teaspoon dried marjoram
½ teaspoon dried thyme

Combine all the ingredients in a bowl. Toss to mix well. Stuff into a 10-pound turkey or four Cornish hens.

ONE SERVING
=

100 calories
20 CHO
5 PRO
2 FAT
199 SODIUM
177 POTASSIUM
0 CHOLESTEROL

Exchange Value:
1 Bread Exchange +
1 Vegetable Exchange

TRADITIONAL BREAD DRESSING

(Serves 8)

4 cups bread cubes
1 cup chopped celery
⅓ cup chopped onion
1 tablespoon chopped fresh parsley leaves
1 garlic clove, minced
½ cup hot water *
¼ teaspoon ground black pepper
¼ teaspoon ground sage
¼ teaspoon dried marjoram
¼ teaspoon dried thyme
⅛ teaspoon dried basil

*C*ombine all the ingredients in a large bowl. Toss with a wooden spoon. Pour the mixture into a lightly oiled casserole. Bake in a 350-degree oven for 30 to 40 minutes.

Note: This dressing may also be used as a stuffing for Cornish hens, chicken, and turkey.

ONE SERVING
=
96 calories
20 CHO
5 PRO
2 FAT
198 SODIUM
161 POTASSIUM
0 CHOLESTEROL

Exchange Value:
1 Bread Exchange +
1 Vegetable Exchange

---

* For a more moist dressing, use ¾ cup warm water.

CRANBERRY–RICE STUFFING

(Serves 4)

¼ cup brown rice, uncooked
¾ cup water
1 tablespoon vegetable oil
1½ cups sliced mushrooms (½ pound)
½ cup chopped celery
¼ cup chopped onion
1 cup fresh or frozen cranberries
¼ teaspoon dried thyme
¼ teaspoon dried basil

ONE SERVING
=
88 calories
11 CHO
2 PRO
4 FAT
82 SODIUM
172 POTASSIUM
0 CHOLESTEROL

Cook the rice in the water until tender, about 1 hour. Sauté the remaining ingredients in a skillet until the celery and onion are tender. Add the rice and stir to blend. Use as a stuffing in two Cornish hens or one small chicken.

Exchange Value:
½ Bread Exchange
+ ½ Fruit Exchange
+ 1 Fat Exchange

WILD RICE–PINE NUT STUFFING

(Serves 2)

¼ cup wild rice, uncooked
1 cup water
1 green onion (scallion)
1 small garlic clove, minced
1 teaspoon vegetable oil
¼ cup pine nuts, lightly toasted
½ teaspoon dried thyme

ONE SERVING
=
182 calories
15 CHO
4 PRO
11 FAT
138 SODIUM
114 POTASSIUM
0 CHOLESTEROL

Exchange Value:
1 Bread Exchange +
2 Fat Exchanges

Cook the wild rice in the water until tender, about 1 hour. Add more water, if needed.

Meanwhile, sauté the onion, garlic, pine nuts, and thyme in the oil. Add the wild rice. Simmer for 10 minutes to blend the flavors. Cool enough to stuff into quail or one Cornish hen.

CRANBERRY–WILD RICE STUFFING

(Serves 4)

½ cup wild rice, uncooked
1 cup water
¼ cup dark or golden raisins
5 green onions (scallions), chopped
1 tablespoon vegetable oil
½ cup chopped celery or fennel bulb
1 cup fresh or frozen cranberries
1 teaspoon grated orange rind
½ teaspoon dried thyme

ONE SERVING
=
162 calories
24 CHO
2 PRO
7 FAT
147 SODIUM
158 POTASSIUM
0 CHOLESTEROL

Exchange Value:
1 Bread Exchange +
1 Fruit Exchange +
1 Fat Exchange

*P*ut the wild rice in a saucepan. Add the water and raisins and cook over medium heat for 1 hour, or until the rice is tender. Drain.

Sauté the onions and celery (or fennel bulb) in the oil until tender. Add the cranberries, orange rind, thyme, and rice. Stuff into two Cornish hens or a 3-pound chicken, or use with turkey breast. Bake in a 350-degree oven for 1 hour, or until the poultry is done.

APPLE AND PRUNE DRESSING

(Serves 16)

¼ cup vegetable oil
1 medium-size onion
2 celery stalks, cored and chopped
2 apples, chopped
16 prunes, snipped into pieces
1 cup water
10 slices fresh whole wheat bread cubes (6 cups)
1 teaspoon dried sage, crushed
¼ teaspoon ground cinnamon

*C*ombine the oil, onion, celery, and apples in a large skillet. Sauté for about 10 minutes, or until the vegetables are tender. Remove from the heat. Add the remaining ingredients. Toss gently to mix well. Use to stuff a 12- to 18-pound turkey or spoon the stuffing mixture into an oiled 2-quart baking dish. When baking the stuffing in a casserole, cover and bake in a 325-degree oven for about 1 hour.

ONE SERVING
=
100 calories
16 CHO
2 PRO
4 FAT
79 SODIUM
140 POTASSIUM
0 CHOLESTEROL

Exchange Value:
½ Bread Exchange
+ ½ Fruit Exchange
+ 1 Fat Exchange

APRICOT DRESSING
FOR TURKEY

(Serves 12)

1 cup dried apricots, snipped (measure before
   snipping)
1½ cups water or chicken or turkey stock
1 cup chopped celery
¼ cup chopped walnuts or pine nuts
12 slices whole wheat or white bread, dried or toasted
   and cut into small cubes

*B*ring the apricots and water (or chicken or turkey
stock) just to a boil in a saucepan. Let stand for 10
minutes. Add the celery, nuts, and bread. Toss lightly
to moisten the bread and blend the ingredients. Spoon
into an oiled baking dish with a cover. Bake in a 350-
degree oven for about 40 minutes. Remove the cover
for the last 10 minutes of baking to brown the top of
the dressing.

**ONE
SERVING**
=
118 calories
22 CHO
4 PRO
3 FAT
127 SODIUM
215 POTASSIUM
0 CHOLESTEROL

Exchange Value:
1 Bread Exchange +
½ Fat Exchange +
½ Fruit Exchange

RICE AND LENTILS
(Serves 4)

1 medium-size onion, chopped
2 garlic cloves, minced
2 tablespoons vegetable oil
1 teaspoon ground turmeric
½ teaspoon paprika
¼ teaspoon ground cloves
¼ teaspoon ground cinnamon
¼ teaspoon ground coriander
¼ teaspoon ground black pepper
¼ teaspoon salt
1 cup brown rice, uncooked
1 cup dried lentils, sorted and washed
4 cups water

ONE SERVING
=
232 calories
34 CHO
10 PRO
8 FAT
262 SODIUM
325 POTASSIUM
0 CHOLESTEROL

Exchange Value:
2 Bread Exchanges
+ 1 Lean Meat
Exchange + 1 Fat
Exchange

Sauté the onion and garlic in the oil in a large saucepan. Add the spices and cook over low heat for 4 minutes. Add the rice and lentils and stir to mix well. Pour in the water. Bring to a boil, turn the heat to low, and cook for 45 to 50 minutes, or until the rice and lentils are tender.

TOFU FIESTA

(Serves 2)

¼ cup chopped onion
1 garlic clove, minced
1 tablespoon vegetable oil
1 cup broccoli pieces
2 carrots, sliced thin
½ sweet green pepper, sliced thin
1½ cups diced mushrooms
1 cup chopped celery
8 ounces tofu, drained
½ teaspoon ground turmeric
½ cup ricotta cheese
1 ripe tomato, cubed
2 tablespoons chopped fresh parsley leaves
2 tablespoons sesame seeds, toasted

*S*auté the onion and garlic in the oil until the onion is transparent. Add the broccoli, carrots, pepper, mushrooms, and celery and cook until tender. Break the tofu into chunks. Add the tofu to the vegetables with the turmeric and cheese. Simmer to heat thoroughly. Just before serving, add the tomato and parsley and sprinkle on the sesame seeds.

**ONE
SERVING**
=
383 calories
25 CHO
23 PRO
23 FAT
149 SODIUM
1090 POTASSIUM
31 CHOLESTEROL

Exchange Value:
1 Bread Exchange +
2 Vegetable
Exchanges + 2
Medium-Fat Meat
Exchanges + 2 Fat
Exchanges

AFRICAN VEGETARIAN STEW

(Serves 8)

4 small kohlrabies, peeled and cut into chunks
1 large onion, chopped
2 sweet potatoes, peeled and cut into chunks
2 zucchini, sliced thick
5 fresh or 1 16-ounce can tomatoes
1 15-ounce can garbanzo beans (chick-peas) with liquid
½ cup couscous or bulgar wheat
¼ cup dark or golden raisins
1 teaspoon ground coriander
½ teaspoon ground turmeric
½ teaspoon ground cinnamon
½ teaspoon ground ginger
¼ teaspoon ground cumin
3 cups water

ONE SERVING
=
241 calories
42 CHO
8 PRO
2 FAT
22 SODIUM
658 POTASSIUM
0 CHOLESTEROL

Exchange Value:
2 Bread Exchanges
+ 2 Vegetable
Exchanges

Combine all the ingredients in a large saucepan. Bring to a boil, lower the heat, and simmer until the vegetables are tender, about 30 minutes.

Note: Serve the couscous separately, if desired. Parsnips may be substituted for the kohlrabi.

STUFFED CHEESE PIZZA

(Serves 8)

1 package (or 1 tablespoon) active dry yeast
¼ cup warm water (110 to 115 degrees)
3 cups whole wheat flour
½ teaspoon salt
1 tablespoon dried oregano
2 tablespoons vegetable oil
1 cup water
3 cups grated part skim mozzarella cheese
1 10-ounce package frozen broccoli spears, defrosted
    and chopped, OR 2 cups cooked fresh broccoli,
    chopped
1 cup pizza sauce

*T*o make the crust, dissolve the yeast in the warm water in a large bowl. Add the flour, salt, oregano, oil, and 1 cup water. Mix well. Knead the dough on a lightly floured surface for about 2 minutes, or until the dough is smooth. Place the dough in an oiled bowl. Cover with a damp towel and let rise in a warm place for 1 hour, or until doubled in bulk. Punch down the dough. Divide into two parts. Press half the dough onto the bottom of a 10-inch oiled pie pan. Sprinkle the cheese and broccoli over the dough. Press the other half of the dough into a 10-inch round. Set on top of the cheese and broccoli. Crimp the edges together. Make several slashes in the top crust. Bake in a 400-degree oven for 20 to 25 minutes, or until golden brown. Remove from the oven. Spread on the pizza sauce. Bake for 5 minutes.

**ONE
SERVING**
=
282 calories
37 CHO
16 PRO
10 FAT
424 SODIUM
425 POTASSIUM
16 CHOLESTEROL

Exchange Value:
2 Medium-Fat Meat
Exchanges + 2
Bread Exchanges +
2 Vegetable
Exchanges

WHOLE WHEAT PIZZA

(Serves 8)

1 cup warm water (110 to 115 degrees)
1 package (or 1 tablespoon) active dry yeast OR 1 cake
  yeast
1 tablespoon honey
1 cup whole wheat flour
½ teaspoon salt
1 tablespoon vegetable oil
4 ounces Cheddar cheese, grated
½ teaspoon ground black pepper
½ teaspoon caraway seeds
¼ teaspoon garlic powder
1¼ to 1½ cups whole wheat flour
½ cup tomato sauce or pizza sauce
½ to 1 tablespoon dried oregano
1 cup raw broccoli pieces
1 cup raw zucchini slices
1 cup raw mushroom slices
8 ounces part skim mozzarella cheese, shredded

ONE SERVING
=

305 calories
33 CHO
18 PRO
12 FAT
430 SODIUM
378 POTASSIUM
31 CHOLESTEROL

Exchange Value:
2 Medium-Fat Meat
Exchanges + 2
Bread Exchanges +
1 Vegetable Exchange

Combine the water, yeast, honey, and the 1 cup of whole wheat flour in a large bowl. Beat 100 times until mixture is smooth. Let rise in a warm place for 15 minutes. Add the salt, oil, Cheddar cheese, pepper, caraway seeds, garlic powder, and 1¼ to 1½ cups whole wheat flour. Mix well and let the dough rest for 5 minutes. Pat out the dough onto a baking sheet for 1 large pizza or divide the dough in half and make two medium-size pizzas. Top with the pizza sauce, oregano, vegetables, and mozzarella. Bake in a 400-degree oven for 15 to 20 minutes.

BRUNCH PIZZA

(Serves 6)

Pizza crust, prepared or homemade
½ pound boiled ham, sliced
8 ounces part skim mozzarella cheese, grated
2 eggs
¼ cup lowfat milk
Pinch of dried oregano

*P*at the pizza dough out on a 13- by 9-inch pan, baking sheet, or a round pizza pan. Cut the ham into strips and put them on the dough. Sprinkle on the cheese. Combine the eggs and milk in a bowl and beat to blend. Pour the eggs over the dough and sprinkle on the oregano. Bake in a 375-degree oven for 20 to 30 minutes.

**ONE
SERVING**
=
277 calories
15 CHO
19 PRO
15 FAT
785 SODIUM
206 POTASSIUM
145 CHOLESTEROL

Exchange Value:
1 Bread Exchange + 2
Medium-Fat Meat
Exchanges + 1 Fat
Exchange

CHEESE AND RICE CASSEROLE

(Serves 4)

2½ cups brown rice, cooked
3 green onions (scallions), chopped
1 cup lowfat cottage cheese or hoop cheese
1 teaspoon dried dill
¼ cup grated Parmesan cheese
½ cup lowfat milk

Combine all the ingredients in a mixing bowl. Pour into a lightly oiled casserole. Bake in a 350-degree oven for 15 to 20 minutes.

ONE SERVING
=
235 calories
35 CHO
14 PRO
4 FAT
682 SODIUM
203 POTASSIUM
10 CHOLESTEROL

Exchange Value:
2 Bread Exchanges
+ 1 Lean Meat
Exchange + ½ Milk
Exchange

EGGPLANT–SWISS CHEESE CASSEROLE

(Serves 6)

½ cup chopped onion
1 tablespoon vegetable oil
1 6-ounce can tomato paste
1¾ cups water
2 teaspoons dried oregano
¼ cup chopped fresh parsley leaves OR 2 tablespoons
　dried parsley flakes
½ teaspoon salt
1 large eggplant or zucchini
1 pound Swiss cheese, sliced
1½ cups dry bread cubes
1 cup grated Parmesan cheese

ONE SERVING

=

385 calories
17 CHO
26 PRO
26 FAT
497 SODIUM
471 POTASSIUM
72 CHOLESTEROL

Exchange Value:
3 High-Fat Meat
Exchanges + 1
Bread Exchange + 1
Fat Exchange

Sauté the onion in the oil in a saucepan until the onion is tender. Add the tomato paste, water, oregano, parsley, and salt. Simmer over low heat for 10 minutes. Cut the eggplant (or zucchini) into ¼-inch-thick slices. Arrange one layer of eggplant slices in the bottom of a lightly oiled 9- by 13-inch baking pan. Pour on about ⅓ cup of the tomato sauce. Top with the Swiss cheese slices. Add another layer of eggplant slices and pour on about ½ cup of the tomato sauce. Combine the rest of the sauce with the bread cubes and spoon over the eggplant. Sprinkle on the Parmesan cheese. Bake in a 325-degree oven for about 25 minutes.

8

AROMATIC YEAST BREADS AND COFFEE CAKES

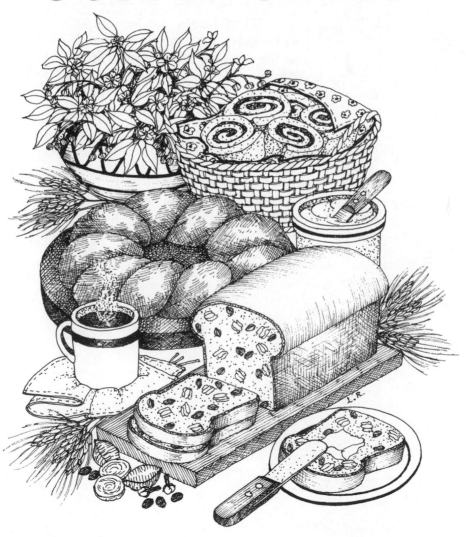

The holidays would not be complete without fresh baked breads and a coffee cake for those special mornings like Christmas and New Year's. Even the busiest of cooks often takes time to make favorite holiday treats.

Note: Although 1 package of yeast measures slightly less than 1 tablespoon, for the purposes of the recipes in this chapter we will consider the two interchangeable. If the yeast is purchased in jars, the 1 tablespoon measurement should be used.

SWEDISH TEA LOG

(Serves 16)

1 package (or 1 tablespoon) active dry yeast
¼ cup warm water (110 to 115 degrees)
1 cup whole wheat flour
1 cup all-purpose flour
2 tablespoons sugar
¼ teaspoon salt
½ cup margarine
¼ cup evaporated lowfat milk
1 egg
½ cup dark or golden raisins
Unsweetened applesauce
Ground cinnamon and nutmeg
Apple slices
Frozen orange juice concentrate

ONE SERVING
=
137 calories
18 CHO
3 PRO
6 FAT
107 SODIUM
110 POTASSIUM
17 CHOLESTEROL

Exchange Value:
1 Bread Exchange +
1 Fat Exchange

*S*often the yeast in the water. Combine the flours, sugar, and salt in a mixing bowl. Cut in the margarine until the mixture resembles crumbs. Add the milk, egg, raisins, and softened yeast and mix well. Cover and chill for 3 hours or overnight.

Divide the dough in half. Roll out half on a floured surface to a 12- by 6-inch rectangle. Spread with ¼ cup applesauce. Sprinkle on cinnamon and nutmeg. Roll up and shape into a crescent on a lightly greased baking sheet. Make cuts along the outside edge about 1 inch apart and to within ½ inch of the center. Then turn each cut at an angle to expose the interior of the roll. Top each cut with a thin slice of apple. Repeat with the remaining dough. Let rise in warm place for about 30 minutes. Bake in a 350-degree oven for 20 to 25 minutes, or until golden brown. Glaze with the orange juice concentrate while still warm.

CHRISTMAS STOLLEN
(Serves 15)

½ cup dark or golden raisins
¼ cup chopped dried apricots
¼ cup unsweetened apple juice or rum
1 package (or 1 tablespoon) active dry yeast
⅓ cup milk, heated to lukewarm (105 to 110 degrees)
½ cup flour
½ cup margarine
2 tablespoons sugar
¼ teaspoon salt
¼ teaspoon almond extract
1 teaspoon grated lemon rind
1 to 1½ cups flour
½ cup sliced blanched almonds
½ cup low sugar apricot preserves

ONE SERVING
=
162 calories
23 CHO
2 PRO
7 FAT
116 SODIUM
121 POTASSIUM
0 CHOLESTEROL

Exchange Value:
1 Bread Exchange +
½ Fruit Exchange +
1 Fat Exchange

Combine the raisins, apricots, and apple juice (or rum) in a bowl. Let soak overnight or for at least 4 hours.

Combine the yeast, milk, and the ½ cup of flour in a bowl. Mix until smooth and the mixture looks like thin mashed potatoes. Cover the bowl with a damp cloth and let rise in a warm place for 10 minutes, or until doubled in bulk.

Meanwhile, cream the margarine, sugar, salt, almond extract, and lemon rind. Beat in the yeast mixture and 1¼ cups of the flour. Turn the dough out onto a lightly floured surface and knead in about ¼ cup more flour, or until the dough is soft. Knead for 3 minutes. Put in a greased bowl, cover with a damp towel, and let rise in a warm place until doubled, about 1½ to 2 hours. Once the dough has doubled, knead in the raisin mixture and almonds. Knead until well mixed. Roll the dough into a rectangular 12- by 6-inch shape. Roll up jelly roll fashion. Place on a lightly oiled baking sheet and let rise about 30 minutes. Bake in a 375-degree oven for 25 to 30 minutes, or until golden brown. Cool partially on a wire rack. Glaze the cool but not cold stollen with the apricot preserves.

PUMPKIN TEA RING

(Serves 25)

1 tablespoon active dry yeast
¼ cup lukewarm water (105 to 110 degrees)
1 cup milk
¼ cup vegetable oil
2 tablespoons sugar
½ teaspoon salt
5 to 5½ cups whole wheat flour
1 16-ounce can pumpkin
1 teaspoon ground cinnamon
½ teaspoon ground nutmeg
¼ teaspoon ground cloves
½ cup currants or dark raisins
2 tablespoons margarine
2 tablespoons honey

ONE SERVING
=
144 calories
25 CHO
4 PRO
4 FAT
17 SODIUM
187 POTASSIUM
0 CHOLESTEROL

Exchange Value:
1 Bread Exchange +
1 Fruit Exchange +
1 Fat Exchange

*S*often the yeast in the water. Combine the milk, oil, sugar, and salt in a large bowl with 2 cups of the flour. Add the yeast mixture, pumpkin, cinnamon, nutmeg, cloves, and currants (or dark raisins). Mix well. Stir in 3 more cups of flour. Beat. Transfer to an oiled bowl, cover with a damp towel, and let rise in a warm place until doubled in bulk, about 1 hour. Punch down the dough and turn onto a lightly floured surface and knead in the remaining flour to make a smooth and elastic dough, about 5 minutes.

Melt the margarine and honey together in a saucepan. Break off 2-inch pieces of dough and shape into balls. Dip them into the honey mixture. Place in an oiled 10-inch tube pan. Cover and let rise in a warm place until doubled, about 1 hour. Bake in a 350-degree oven for 50 to 60 minutes. Let cool for 10 minutes before removing from the pan. Serve warm.

APRICOT KOLACHY

(Serves 24)

1 tablespoon active dry yeast
¼ cup lukewarm water (105 to 110 degrees)
¼ cup plus 2 tablespoons sugar
¼ cup margarine
½ teaspoon salt
2 eggs
½ teaspoon lemon extract
1 cup water
3½ to 4 cups flour
24 dried apricots or prunes
½ teaspoon ground cinnamon

ONE SERVING
=
114 calories
20 CHO
3 PRO
3 FAT
79 SODIUM
81 POTASSIUM
23 CHOLESTEROL

Exchange Value:
1 Bread Exchange +
½ Fat Exchange +
½ Fruit Exchange

*D*issolve the yeast in the ¼ cup of lukewarm water. Add the ¼ cup sugar and margarine. When the margarine is soft, add the salt, eggs, lemon extract, ½ cup of water, and 3 cups of the flour. Beat until thoroughly blended. Place on a floured surface and knead in extra flour to make a soft, smooth dough. Transfer to a lightly oiled bowl, cover with a damp towel, and let rise in a warm place until doubled, about 1 hour.

Meanwhile, cook the apricots in the remaining ½ cup of water for 15 to 20 minutes, or until softened. Purée in a blender. Add the cinnamon and the remaining 2 tablespoons of sugar and mix well. Cool until needed.

Punch the dough down and let it rest for 5 minutes. Roll out on a floured surface to approximately ½ inch thick and cut into 2-inch circles. Place a spoonful of the apricot (or prune) filling in the center. Place on an oiled baking sheet. Let rise for 15 minutes. Bake in a 400-degree oven for 10 to 15 minutes, or until browned.

FIG SQUARE

(Serves 16)

1 package (or 1 tablespoon) active dried yeast
¼ cup warm water (110 to 115 degrees)
¼ cup sugar
½ teaspoon salt
2 tablespoons vegetable oil
½ cup milk at room temperature
1 egg
1 teaspoon grated orange rind
1 cup whole wheat flour
1¼ cups unbleached white flour
1½ cups snipped dried figs
1 cup water
½ teaspoon ground allspice
confectioners sugar (optional)

ONE SERVING
=
136 calories
26 CHO
3 PRO
3 FAT
72 SODIUM
164 POTASSIUM
17 CHOLESTEROL

Exchange Value:
1 Bread Exchange +
1 Fruit Exchange +
½ Fat Exchange

*S*often the yeast in the warm water. Combine the sugar, salt, oil, milk, egg, and orange rind in a large bowl. Beat well. Add the yeast mixture and the 1 cup of whole wheat flour. Beat. Add the remaining flour. Extra flour may be needed if the dough is sticky. Turn onto a lightly floured surface and knead until smooth, about 5 minutes. Transfer to an oiled bowl, cover with a damp towel, and let rise for 1 hour.

Meanwhile, prepare the fig filling by combining the figs, water, and allspice in a saucepan. Bring to a boil, lower the heat, and simmer until the mixture is thick. Mash the figs with a potato masher or large spoon during cooking. Cool.

Punch down the dough. Roll into a ½-inch-thick rectangle 8 inches wide. Spread with the fig filling. Roll up like a jelly roll. Fit into a lightly oiled 8-inch-square pan. Seal the edges together. At each corner, cut with a scissors to fit into the shape of the pan. Make two slashes on top of each side. Let rise until doubled, about 30 minutes. Bake in a 350-degree oven for 20 to 25 minutes. Cool. May be sprinkled lightly with confectioners sugar just before serving.

SAFFRON BREAD

(Serves 15)

½ teaspoon saffron
¼ cup hot water (120 to 130 degrees)
1 cup milk
¼ cup margarine
1 tablespoon grated lemon rind
1 tablespoon active dry yeast
¼ cup sugar
¼ teaspoon ground nutmeg
2½ to 3 cups flour
1 cup dried currants or dark raisins

ONE SERVING
=
160 calories
20 CHO
3 PRO
3 FAT
46 SODIUM
132 POTASSIUM
0 CHOLESTEROL

Exchange Value:
1 Bread Exchange +
½ Fruit Exchange +
½ Fat Exchange

Steep the saffron in the hot water for 10 to 15 minutes.

Meanwhile, combine the milk and margarine in a saucepan. Heat until the margarine has melted. Cool. Add the lemon rind. Sprinkle the yeast into the milk mixture when lukewarm. Let stand for 5 minutes to dissolve. Add the sugar, nutmeg, 2 cups of the flour, and the saffron mixture. Beat until smooth. Stir in the currants (or dark raisins) and another ½ cup of the flour. Cover with a damp towel and let rise in a warm place until doubled in size. Then punch down and knead on a lightly floured board until smooth.

Shape into a loaf and place in an oiled 4- by 9-inch bread pan. Let rise until doubled. Bake in a 350-degree oven for about 1 hour. Cool for 10 minutes in the pan before turning out on a wire rack. When the bread is thoroughly cooled, it may be sliced.

SWEDISH CARDAMOM BRAID

(Serves 12)

2 tablespoons active dry yeast
½ cup lukewarm water (105 to 110 degrees)
½ cup milk, scalded
¼ cup sugar
½ teaspoon salt
¼ cup vegetable oil
1 egg
3½ to 4 cups flour
1 teaspoon ground cardamom
½ cup dark or golden raisins

ONE SERVING
=
121 calories
17 CHO
2 PRO
5 FAT
94 SODIUM
89 POTASSIUM
23 CHOLESTEROL

Exchange Value:
1 Bread Exchange +
1 Fat Exchange

Combine the yeast and the lukewarm water. Let stand until dissolved. Pour the hot milk over the sugar to dissolve it. Add the salt and vegetable oil. Cool. Stir in the yeast mixture, egg, 3 cups of the flour, and the cardamom into the sugar mixture. Add the raisins and extra flour. Beat until smooth. Turn the dough onto a lightly floured surface. Knead until smooth and elastic. Transfer to a lightly oiled bowl, cover with a damp towel, and let rise in a warm place until doubled, about 1 hour. Punch down the dough and transfer to a lightly floured surface. Divide into thirds. Roll each part into a 10-inch-long strand. Braid loosely. Place on a lightly oiled baking sheet. Cover and let rise in a warm place until doubled, about 1 hour. Bake in a 350-degree oven for 30 to 35 minutes.

HOLIDAY CRANBERRY ROLLS

(Serves 18)

1 package (or 1 tablespoon) active dry yeast
¼ cup warm water (110 to 115 degrees)
1 cup whole wheat flour
1½ cups unbleached all-purpose flour
1 tablespoon sugar
¼ teaspoon salt
½ cup lowfat milk
2 eggs

Cranberry–Orange Filling
  1½ cups fresh or frozen cranberries
  1 orange, peeled
  2 tablespoons dark or light brown sugar or fructose
  ¼ cup unsweetened applesauce
  Frozen orange juice concentrate

ONE SERVING
=
140 calories
19 CHO
3 PRO
6 FAT
99 SODIUM
92 POTASSIUM
31 CHOLESTEROL

Exchange Value:
1 Bread Exchange +
1 Fat Exchange

Soften the yeast in the warm water. Combine the flours, sugar, and salt in a mixing bowl. Cut in the margarine until the mixture resembles crumbs. Add the milk, eggs, and softened yeast. Mix well. Cover and refrigerate for 2 hours or overnight.

Meanwhile, make the Cranberry–Orange Filling by combining the cranberries, orange, brown sugar (or fructose), and applesauce in a food procesor. Grind until coarse. Transfer to a saucepan and cook over medium heat for 10 minutes. Cool.

After chilling, roll the dough into an 18- by 12-inch rectangle on a floured surface. Spread with the filling. Roll up jelly roll fashion. Cut into 18 rolls with a sharp knife. Place in an oiled 13- by 9-inch baking pan. Let rise in a warm place for about 30 minutes, or until doubled in bulk. Bake in a 350-degree oven for 25 to 30 minutes, or until golden brown. Glaze with orange juice concentrate while still warm.

WHOLE WHEAT–PECAN ROLLS

(Serves 16)

1 package (or 1 tablespoon) active dry yeast
½ cup warm water (110 to 115 degrees)
⅓ cup skim milk
1 tablespoon dark or light brown sugar
½ teaspoon salt
¼ cup vegetable oil
1 cup unbleached white flour
1 to 1½ cups whole wheat flour
¼ cup dark or golden raisins
1 tablespoon margarine
1 teaspoon ground cinnamon
2 tablespoons honey
¼ cup chopped pecans

ONE SERVING
=
136 calories
19 CHO
3 PRO
6 FAT
76 SODIUM
85 POTASSIUM
0 CHOLESTEROL

Exchange Value:
1 Bread Exchange +
1 Fat Exchange

Soften the yeast in the warm water in a large bowl. Add the milk, sugar, salt, and vegetable oil. Stir to blend. Add the white flour, 1¼ cups of the whole wheat flour, and the raisins. Beat well. More whole wheat flour may be added to make a stiff dough. Transfer the dough to a lightly floured board or counter and knead 2 to 3 minutes to develop the gluten. Put the dough in a lightly oiled bowl. Cover with a damp towel and let rise in a warm place for 40 minutes, or until doubled in bulk.

Transfer to a lightly floured surface and roll into a 16- by 6-inch rectangle. Spread with 1 tablespoon margarine. Sprinkle on the cinnamon. Roll up the dough. Spread the honey and nuts evenly over the bottom of an oiled 9-inch-square pan. Cut the dough into 1-inch pieces and put them in the pan. Let rise about 20 minutes, or until doubled in bulk. Bake in a 375-degree oven for 15 to 20 minutes.

OATMEAL–BRAN BREAD

(Serves 30)

1 cup oatmeal
2 cups water
¼ cup dark or light molasses
2 tablespoons vegetable oil
½ teaspoon salt
1 package (or 1 tablespoon) active dry yeast
½ cup warm water (110 to 115 degrees)
1 cup bran
¼ cup soy flour
½ cup wheat germ
3 cups whole wheat flour

ONE SERVING
=
79 calories
14 CHO
3 PRO
2 FAT
44 SODIUM
154 POTASSIUM
0 CHOLESTEROL

Exchange Value:
1 Bread Exchange

Cook the oatmeal according to directions in the 2 cups of water. Add the molasses, oil, and salt. Cool to lukewarm. Dissolve the yeast in the warm water and add to the oatmeal mixture. Stir in the bran, soy flour, and wheat germ. Beat in the whole wheat flour, adding a little at a time, until the dough is stiff. Knead the dough on a floured surface until it is smooth and elastic. Cover with a damp towel and let rise in a warm place in a lightly oiled bowl until doubled in bulk. Punch down and knead again until smooth and elastic.

Divide the dough into two loaves. Shape and put into lightly oiled bread pans. Let rise until doubled. Bake in a 375-degree oven for about 40 minutes, or until brown and sounds hollow when tapped on top. Remove from the pan immediately and cool on a wire rack.

GREEK CHRISTMAS BREAD

(Serves 15)

1 package (or 1 tablespoon) active dry yeast
¼ cup warm water (110 to 115 degrees)
⅓ cup sugar
1 teaspoon ground cardamom
¼ teaspoon salt
1 egg
¼ cup milk
¼ cup vegetable oil
1½ cups whole wheat flour
1 cup all-purpose flour
¼ cup golden raisins
¼ cup chopped walnuts

ONE SERVING

=

147 calories
22 CHO
4 PRO
6 FAT
40 SODIUM
101 POTASSIUM
18 CHOLESTEROL

Exchange Value:
1 Bread Exchange +
½ Fruit Exchange +
1 Fat Exchange

Dissolve the yeast in the warm water. Combine the sugar, cardamom, salt, egg, milk, and oil in a large bowl. Mix well. Add the yeast mixture, flours, raisins, and nuts. Mix well. Add enough extra flour to make soft dough. Turn the dough out onto a floured surface and knead until smooth and elastic, about 5 minutes. Shape into a round loaf.

Put the dough into a lightly oiled 8-inch-round cake pan. Cover with a damp towel and let rise in a warm place until doubled in bulk, about 1 hour. Bake in a 350-degree oven 35 to 40 minutes, or until brown.

YUGOSLAVIAN CHRISTMAS BREAD "POTIKA"
(Serves 15)

¾ cup milk
¼ cup sugar
1 package (or 1 tablespoon) active dry yeast
½ cup unbleached all-purpose flour
1 cup whole wheat flour
¼ teaspoon salt
2 tablespoons vegetable oil
1 egg
½ cup chopped walnuts
2 ounces semisweet chocolate, grated, OR 1 ounce
   unsweetened chocolate plus 1 teaspoon sugar

*H*eat the milk to 105 degrees. Cool. Add the 1
teaspoon of sugar and yeast. Stir to dissolve. Set aside
until foamy, about 5 minutes.

Combine the flours, ¼ cup sugar, salt, oil, and egg in
a mixing bowl. Beat in the milk mixture. Mix well.
Transfer the dough to a lightly floured board; knead
for 2 minutes, or until smooth and elastic. Shape into a
ball and place in a lightly oiled bowl. Cover with a
damp towel and let rise in a warm place for 30 to 45
minutes, or until doubled.

Meanwhile, combine the nuts and chocolate in a
bowl.

When the dough has doubled, punch it down and
roll into a ¼-inch-thick rectangle. Spread the chocolate–
nut mixture over the dough. Roll up jelly roll style.
Place the roll on a lightly oiled baking pan or in a 9- by
5-inch bread pan. Cover with a damp towel and let rise
in a warm place for 20 to 30 minutes. Bake in a 350-
degree oven for 30 to 40 minutes. Cool on a wire rack.

**ONE
SERVING**
=
124 calories
14 CHO
3 PRO
7 FAT
44 SODIUM
104 POTASSIUM
19 CHOLESTEROL

Exchange Value:
1 Bread Exchange +
1 Fat Exchange

HOLIDAY FRUIT AND NUT BREAD

(Serves 25)

2 cups snipped dried apricots (½ pound)
1½ cups dried currants (¼ pound)
½ cup snipped dried dates
½ cup chopped pecans
1¼ cups water
½ cup apricot brandy or unsweetened apple juice
1 package (or 1 tablespoon) active dry yeast
¼ cup warm water (110 to 115 degrees)
½ cup vegetable oil
¼ cup honey
½ teaspoon ground cinnamon
¼ teaspoon ground cloves
1 cup unbleached pastry flour
2 to 2¼ cups whole wheat flour

ONE SERVING
=
164 calories
26 CHO
3 PRO
8 FAT
2 SODIUM
224 POTASSIUM
0 CHOLESTEROL

Exchange Value:
1 Bread Exchange +
1 Fruit Exchange +
1 Fat Exchange

*C*ombine the apricots, currants, dates, pecans, 1¼ cups water, and brandy in a bowl. Let stand overnight or for at least 3 hours. Dissolve the yeast in the warm water. Add the oil, honey, cinnamon, and cloves. Blend in the dried fruit and nut mixture. Stir in enough pastry flour and whole wheat flour to make a stiff dough. Beat well. Spoon the dough into two 5- by seven-inch bread pans. Cover with a damp towel and let rise in a warm place for 1 to 1½ hours, or until almost doubled. Bake in a 400-degree oven for 30 to 40 minutes. Cool in the pan for 10 minutes. Remove and cool completely on a wire rack. When cooled thoroughly, wrap in aluminum foil and store for at least 3 days before serving. Bread may be made several weeks ahead and kept in an airtight container in a cool place.

PEAR TEA RING

(Serves 25)

2 cups (½ pound) snipped dried pears
1½ cups dark or golden raisins or dried currants
   (¼ pound)
¾ cup snipped dried figs (⅛ pound)
¾ cup chopped walnuts
2 cups water
⅓ cup brandy or unsweetened apple juice
1 package (or 1 tablespoon) active dry yeast
¼ cup warm water (110 to 115 degrees)
⅓ cup vegetable oil
⅓ cup sugar
¾ teaspoon ground cinnamon
3¾ to 4 cups whole wheat flour

ONE SERVING
=
190 calories
34 CHO
4 PRO
6 FAT
3 SODIUM
249 POTASSIUM
0 CHOLESTEROL

Exchange Value:
1 Bread Exchange +
1½ Fruit Exchanges
+ 1 Fat Exchange

Combine the pears, raisins (or dried currants), figs, walnuts, 2 cups water, and brandy (or unsweetened apple juice) in a bowl. Let stand overnight or at least 3 hours. Dissolve the yeast in the warm water. Add the oil, sugar, and cinnamon. Blend in the dried fruit and nut mixture. Stir in enough flour to make a stiff dough. Beat well. Spoon the dough into a 10-inch tube pan or Bundt pan. Let rise in a warm place 1 to 1½ hours, or until almost doubled. Bake in a 400-degree oven for 30 to 40 minutes. Cool in the pan for 10 minutes. Remove from the pan and cool completely on a wire rack. When cooled thoroughly, wrap in aluminum foil and store for at least 3 days before serving. Cake may be kept in an airtight container in a cool place for several weeks before use.

PINEAPPLE–CARROT COFFEE RING

(Serves 16)

1 package (or 1 tablespoon) active dry yeast
¼ cup warm water (110 to 115 degrees)
1 egg
2 tablespoons honey
1 cup unbleached white flour
1 8-ounce can crushed pineapple in its own juice
1 cup grated carrots (2 medium)
¼ cup dark or golden raisins
¼ teaspoon salt
½ teaspoon ground cinnamon
¼ teaspoon ground nutmeg
¼ cup sunflower seeds
1½ cups whole wheat flour
½ cup bran
2 tablespoons vegetable oil

ONE SERVING
=
130 calories
22 CHO
4 PRO
4 FAT
41 SODIUM
174 POTASSIUM
17 CHOLESTEROL

Exchange Value:
1 Bread Exchange +
½ Fruit Exchange +
1 Fat Exchange

Sprinkle the yeast over the warm water in a bowl. Stir to dissolve the yeast. Combine the egg, honey, yeast mixture, unbleached white flour, and pineapple in a mixing bowl. Beat well. Let stand in a warm place for 30 minutes covered with a wet towel. Add the carrots, raisins, salt, cinnamon, nutmeg, sunflower seeds, whole wheat flour, bran, and oil. Blend well. Spoon the dough into a lightly oiled 10-inch tube pan. Let rise until doubled in a warm place for 60 minutes. Bake in a 350-degree oven for 25 minutes, or until browned. Cool in the pan for 5 minutes; then remove from the pan and cool completely on a wire rack.

NO-KNEAD BRAN BREAD

(Serves 18)

3 cups whole wheat flour
½ cup dry milk powder
½ teaspoon salt
2 tablespoons active dry yeast
¼ cup honey
1¼ cups warm water (110 to 115 degrees)
1½ cups bran OR 2 cups bran cereal
1 egg
3 tablespoons vegetable oil

ONE SERVING
=
128 calories
22 CHO
4 PRO
4 FAT
66 SODIUM
167 POTASSIUM
15 CHOLESTEROL

Exchange Value:
1 Bread Exchange +
1 Fat Exchange

Stir together the flour, dry milk powder, and salt. Combine the yeast, honey, warm water, and bran in a large mixing bowl. Let the yeast mixture stand 2 minutes. Add the egg, oil, and about half of the flour mixture. Beat until smooth. Add the remaining flour mixture and stir to form a sticky dough. Cover with a damp towel and let rise in a warm place until doubled in bulk, about 1 hour. Stir down and pour into a lightly greased 9- by 5-inch loaf pan. Bake in a 375-degree oven for about 40 minutes. Cool in the pan for 5 minutes. Remove and cool thoroughly on a wire rack.

WHOLE WHEAT BREAD

(Serves 26)

¾ cup skim milk
2 tablespoons sugar
2 teaspoons salt
⅓ cup vegetable oil
⅓ cup light or dark molasses
1½ cups warm water (110 to 115 degrees)
2 tablespoons active dry yeast
4½ cups whole wheat flour
2 cups unbleached white flour

ONE SERVING

=

105 calories
19 CHO
3 PRO
2 FAT
115 SODIUM
128 POTASSIUM
0 CHOLESTEROL

Exchange Value:
1 Bread Exchange

Scald the milk and stir in the sugar, salt, oil, and molasses. Cool to lukewarm.

Meanwhile, combine the warm water and yeast in a mixing bowl and stir until the yeast is dissolved. Stir in the milk mixture. Add 2 cups of the whole wheat flour and 1 cup of the unbleached flour. Beat until smooth. Stir in the remaining flours. Turn the dough onto a lightly floured surface. Knead until smooth and elastic. Place in a greased bowl. Brush the top with vegetable oil. Cover with a damp towel and let rise in a warm place for about 1 hour, or until doubled. Turn onto a lightly floured board. Divide in half. Shape into loaves. Place in lightly oiled 9- by 5- by 3-inch bread pans. Cover and let rise in a warm place until doubled, about 1 hour. Bake in a 400-degree oven for about 45 minutes.

9

HOLIDAY DESSERTS

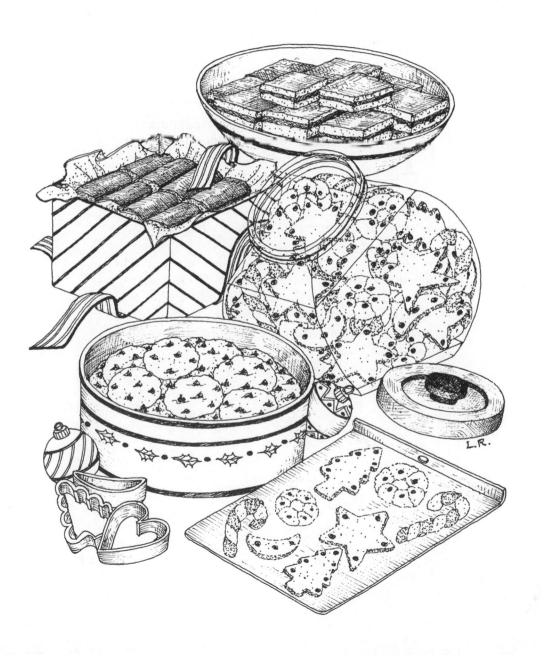

Fruitcake and cookies are holiday traditions in many homes. Dried fruits, such as apricots, prunes, and dates are better sources of nutrition than the chopped candied fruit that is added to most fruitcake recipes. Orange juice and grated orange rind are used to replace citron in traditional fruitcake recipes.

Holiday bar cookies and rolled cookies add variety to dessert selections. These cookies can be made ahead of the busy holiday season and frozen. To thaw the cookies, place them on a baking sheet or wire rack at room temperature for 2 to 3 hours.

FRUIT AND NUT BALLS

(Serves 12)

½ cup pitted dates
½ cup dark or golden raisins
2 tablespoons cocoa or carob powder
½ cup walnuts
½ cup sunflower seeds
Ground walnuts

Grind together dates, raisins, cocoa (or carob powder), walnuts, and sunflower seeds in a food processor or meat grinder. Press the mixture into 24 small balls. Roll in the ground nuts. Store in an airtight container.

TWO BALLS
=
94 calories
10 CHO
2 PRO
6 FAT
2 SODIUM
101 POTASSIUM
0 CHOLESTEROL

Exchange Value:
1 Fruit Exchange +
1 Fat Exchange

RUSSIAN TEA CAKES

(Makes 36)

1 cup margarine, softened
¼ cup confectioners sugar
1 teaspoon vanilla extract
2 cups flour
½ cup chopped pecans, toasted
Confectioners sugar

Cream the margarine, sugar, and vanilla together until light and fluffy. Mix in the flour and pecans. Chill for 2 hours. Pinch off small pieces of dough and roll into 1-inch balls. Place on an ungreased baking sheet. Bake in a 375-degree oven until very lightly brown, 10 to 12 minutes. Cool on a wire rack. Roll in confectioners sugar before serving. Store in an airtight container.

ONE CAKE
=
84 calories
6 CHO
1 PRO
6 FAT
59 SODIUM
19 POTASSIUM
0 CHOLESTEROL

Exchange Value:
½ Bread Exchange
+ 1 Fat Exchange

APPLESAUCE–RAISIN COOKIES

(Makes 24)

¼ cup vegetable oil
¼ cup sugar
1 egg
1 teaspoon vanilla extract
½ cup unsweetened applesauce
½ cup whole wheat flour
½ cup unbleached white flour
2 teaspoons baking powder
½ teaspoon baking soda
1 teaspoon ground cinnamon
⅛ teaspoon ground cloves
½ cup rolled oats
½ cup dark or golden raisins

ONE COOKIE
=
56 calories
10 CHO
1 PRO
2 FAT
47 SODIUM
49 POTASSIUM
11 CHOLESTEROL

Exchange Value:
½ Fruit Exchange +
½ Fat Exchange

*C*ream the oil and sugar together. Add the egg and beat until light. Blend in the vanilla and applesauce. Stir the flours, baking powder, baking soda, cinnamon, cloves, oats, and raisins into the creamed mixture. Blend well. Drop by teaspoonfuls onto lightly oiled baking sheets. Bake in a 375-degree oven for 10 minutes. Cool on a wire rack.

CHRISTMAS FRUITCAKE COOKIES

(Makes 36)

½ cup vegetable oil
½ cup dark or light brown sugar
1 egg
1¼ cups whole wheat flour
½ teaspoon baking powder
1 teaspoon ground cinnamon
¼ teaspoon ground cloves
¼ teaspoon ground allspice
¼ cup milk
½ cup chopped walnuts
½ cup dark or golden raisins
½ cup snipped dried apricots
½ cup chopped dates

ONE COOKIE

=

77 calories
9 CHO
1 PRO
4 FAT
7 SODIUM
70 POTASSIUM
8 CHOLESTEROL

Exchange Value:
½ Fruit Exchange +
1 Fat Exchange

Cream together the oil and sugar. Add the egg. Then blend in the remaining ingredients. Drop by spoonfuls onto a lightly oiled baking sheet. Bake in a 350-degree oven for about 10 minutes. Cool on a wire rack and store in a tightly closed container.

CRANBERRY–ORANGE BARS

(Makes 24)

1 cup finely chopped cranberries (2 cups whole fresh
  or frozen berries)
2 oranges, ground with skins and pulp
½ cup dark or golden raisins
¼ cup dark or light brown sugar*
⅓ cup margarine
2 eggs
1 teaspoon vanilla extract
1 cup whole wheat flour
1 cup unbleached all-purpose flour
2 teaspoons baking powder

ONE BAR
=
86 calories
14 CHO
2 PRO
3 FAT
55 SODIUM
78 POTASSIUM
11 CHOLESTEROL

Exchange Value:
1 Fruit Exchange +
½ Fat Exchange

Combine the cranberries, oranges, raisins, and brown sugar in a mixing bowl. Set aside.

Cream the margarine until light and fluffy. Add 1 egg at a time and beat well. Blend in the vanilla. Gradually add the flours and baking powder to the creamed mixture. Stir in the cranberry mixture and pour the batter into a greased 13- by 9-inch baking pan. Bake in a 350-degree oven for 30 to 40 minutes, or until browned on top. Cool in the pan on a wire rack. Cut into bars.

* 2 tablespoons fructose can be used instead of brown sugar.

PUMPKIN–OATMEAL BARS

(Makes 24)

⅓ cup sugar
½ cup vegetable oil
1 egg
1 cup canned or cooked pumpkin
1½ cups whole wheat flour
3 teaspoons baking powder
½ teaspoon baking soda
¼ teaspoon ground nutmeg
1½ teaspoons ground cinnamon
¼ teaspoon ground cloves
½ cup orange juice
½ cup chopped walnuts
½ cup dark or golden raisins   1½ c. oatmeal
¼ cup coconut

ONE SERVING
=

114 calories
13 CHO
2 PRO
7 FAT
52 SODIUM
104 POTASSIUM
11 CHOLESTEROL

Exchange Value:
1 Bread Exchange +
1 Fat Exchange

*C*ream together the sugar, oil, egg, and pumpkin until light and fluffy. Stir in the flour, baking powder, baking soda, nutmeg, cinnamon, cloves, and orange juice. Add the walnuts and raisins. Stir to blend. Pour into a lightly oiled 13- by 9-inch baking pan. Sprinkle on the coconut. Bake in a 350-degree oven for 25 to 30 minutes. Cool the pan completely on a wire rack for 5 minutes. Cut into bars.

PRUNE–COCONUT BARS

(Makes 16)

2 cups chopped pitted prunes
1 tablespoon grated orange rind
½ cup water
1 cup rolled oats
1 cup whole wheat flour
⅓ cup wheat germ
½ cup coconut, flaked or shredded
½ cup vegetable oil

ONE BAR
=
141 calories
16 CHO
3 PRO
8 FAT
17 SODIUM
145 POTASSIUM
0 CHOLESTEROL

Exchange Value:
1 Bread Exchange +
1½ Fat Exchanges

Cook the prunes, orange rind, and water in a saucepan until the mixture is soft and smooth.

Meanwhile, combine the oats, flour, wheat germ, coconut, and oil in a bowl. Stir to blend. Press half the mixture in the bottom of an 8-inch-square baking pan. Pour the prune mixture on top and spread evenly. Top with the remaining oat mixture and press evenly over the top. Bake in a 350-degree oven for about 30 minutes, or until the topping is lightly browned. Cool in the pan before cutting into bars.

RAISIN BARS

(Makes 16)

1 cup dark or golden raisins
½ cup unsweetened apple juice
1 cup whole wheat flour
½ teaspoon baking soda
1 teaspoon baking powder
1 teaspoon ground cinnamon
¼ teaspoon ground nutmeg
¼ teaspoon ground cloves
1 egg
2 tablespoons vegetable oil
Grated orange rind

ONE BAR
=
76 calories
14 CHO
2 PRO
2 FAT
47 SODIUM
109 POTASSIUM
17 CHOLESTEROL

Exchange Value:
1 Bread Exchange

*I*n a saucepan, combine the raisins and apple juice. Bring to a boil and cool.

Meanwhile, mix the flour, baking soda, baking powder, cinnamon, nutmeg, cloves, egg, and vegetable oil together. Add the raisin mixture and blend thoroughly. Spread the mixture into a lightly oiled 8-inch-square pan. Sprinkle on the grated orange rind. Bake in a 350-degree oven for 30 to 40 minutes. Cool in the pan on a wire rack and cut into bars.

ROLLED SUGAR COOKIES

(Makes 72)

½ cup margarine
½ cup sugar
1 teaspoon vanilla extract
1 egg
2 cups flour
2 teaspoons baking powder

*C*ream together the margarine, sugar, vanilla, and egg until light and fluffy. Add the flour and baking powder. Blend until well mixed. Chill the dough for 2 hours or overnight. Roll out on a lightly floured surface until ⅛ inch thick. Cut with a cookie cutter. Place on an ungreased baking sheet. Bake in a 375-degree oven until lightly browned, about 10 minutes. Cool before storing.

TWO COOKIES
=

58 calories
8 CHO
0 PRO
2 FAT
46 SODIUM
10 POTASSIUM
8 CHOLESTEROL

Exchange Value:
½ Bread Exchange
+ ½ Fat Exchange

10
TEMPTING MUFFINS AND QUICK BREADS

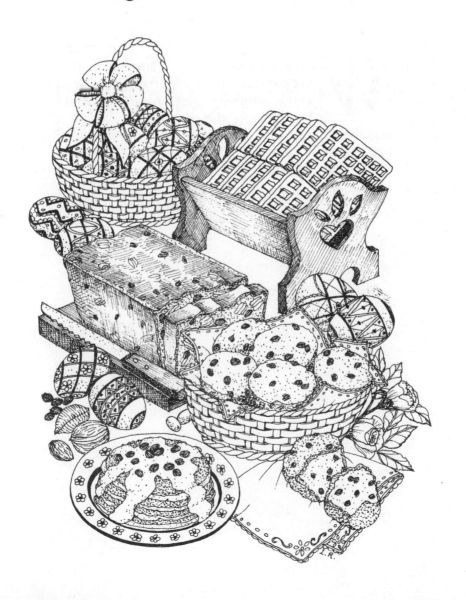

Warm muffins, biscuits, pancakes, and breads are a special treat at any meal. Holiday time means more baking and the aroma of muffins tantalizes the palate. Pumpkin and cranberries are abundant at holiday time and serve as the major flavoring for many of these quick breads.

BRAN MUFFINS

(Makes 6)

¾ cup whole wheat flour
⅓ cup bran
2 teaspoons baking powder
½ teaspoon baking soda
1 tablespoon sugar
2 tablespoons vegetable oil
1 egg
½ cup lowfat milk

ONE MUFFIN
=
128 calories
16 CHO
4 PRO
6 FAT
173 SODIUM
136 POTASSIUM
47 CHOLESTEROL

Exchange Value:
1 Bread Exchange +
1 Fat Exchange

*M*ix the flour, bran, baking powder, baking soda, and sugar in a bowl. Add the oil, egg, and milk. Stir just to combine the ingredients. Spoon into lightly oiled muffin tins. Bake in a 400-degree oven for 15 to 20 minutes.

PEANUT BUTTER–BRAN MUFFINS

(Makes 8)

½ cup whole wheat flour
⅓ cup bran
2 teaspoons baking powder
1 tablespoon sugar
1 egg
¼ cup peanut butter
½ cup lowfat milk
⅓ cup chopped peanuts

ONE MUFFIN
=
140 calories
12 CHO
6 PRO
9 FAT
104 SODIUM
184 POTASSIUM
35 CHOLESTEROL

Exchange Value:
1 Bread Exchange +
2 Fat Exchanges

*C*ombine the flour, bran, baking powder, and sugar in a bowl. Add the remaining ingredients and blend. Spoon into oiled muffin tins or paper muffin cups. Bake in a 375-degree oven for 15 to 20 minutes.

OATMEAL–BANANA MUFFINS

(Makes 12)

3 cups whole wheat flour
¾ cup rolled oats
1 tablespoon baking powder
½ teaspoon ground cinnamon
¼ teaspoon ground nutmeg
1 tablespoon sugar
1 egg
2 tablespoons vegetable oil
½ cup lowfat milk
1 small banana, cubed
¼ cup sunflower seeds, toasted

ONE MUFFIN
=
180 calories
29 CHO
5 PRO
5 FAT
91 SODIUM
221 POTASSIUM
23 CHOLESTEROL

Exchange Value:
1 Bread Exchange +
1 Fruit Exchange +
1 Fat Exchange

Combine the flour, oats, baking powder, cinnamon, nutmeg, and sugar in a bowl. Add the remaining ingredients and blend. Spoon into oiled muffin tins or paper muffin cups. Bake in a 375-degree oven for 15 to 20 minutes.

CRANBERRY–ORANGE MUFFINS

(Makes 6)

½ cup fresh or frozen cranberries
1 egg
½ cup orange juice
1 tablespoon vegetable oil
1 teaspoon grated orange rind
1 cup whole wheat flour
2 teaspoons baking powder
1 tablespoon sugar

*C*ut the cranberries in half and set them aside. Beat together the egg, orange juice, oil, and orange rind. Add the flour, baking powder, and sugar. Stir until all the ingredients are moistened. Add the cranberries. Spoon into oiled muffin tins or paper muffin cups. Bake in a 400-degree oven for 10 to 15 minutes, or until golden brown.

**ONE
MUFFIN**
=
120 calories
20 CHO
4 PRO
3 FAT
95 SODIUM
92 POTASSIUM
46 CHOLESTEROL

Exchange Value:
1 Bread Exchange +
½ Fruit Exchange +
½ Fat Exchange

PUMPKIN–RAISIN MUFFINS
(Makes 8)

1¼ cups whole wheat flour
1 tablespoon sugar or honey
2 teaspoons baking powder
½ teaspoon baking soda
½ teaspoon ground cinnamon
¼ teaspoon ground nutmeg
½ cup orange juice
2 tablespoons vegetable oil
1 egg
½ cup cooked or canned pumpkin
¼ cup dark or golden raisins

ONE MUFFIN
=
105 calories
22 CHO
4 PRO
3 FAT
72 SODIUM
177 POTASSIUM
34 CHOLESTEROL

Exchange Value:
1 Bread Exchange +
½ Fruit Exchange +
½ Fat Exchange

Combine the flour, sugar (or honey), baking powder, baking soda, cinnamon, and nutmeg in a bowl. Mix to blend. Add the orange juice, oil, egg, pumpkin, and raisins. Stir just until the dry ingredients are mixed. Pour into lightly oiled muffin tins. Bake in a 400-degree oven for about 15 minutes.

CORN MUFFINS
(Makes 12)

1 cup cornmeal
1 cup flour
¼ teaspoon salt
3 teaspoons baking powder
1 tablespoon sugar
1 egg
2 tablespoons vegetable oil
¾ cup milk

ONE MUFFIN
=
111 calories
17 CHO
3 PRO
3 FAT
116 SODIUM
53 POTASSIUM
24 CHOLESTEROL

Exchange Value:
1 Bread Exchange +
½ Fat Exchange

Combine all the ingredients in a mixing bowl. Mix to blend. Spoon into lightly oiled muffin tins. Bake in a 400-degree oven for 15 to 20 minutes, or until golden brown.

DILLY RICE MUFFINS
(Makes 8)

1 cup flour
1 tablespoon sugar
1 tablespoon baking powder
1 egg
½ cup lowfat milk
2 tablespoons vegetable oil
¼ cup *cooked* rice
2 tablespoons minced green onion (scallion)
2 tablespoons minced fresh parsley leaves OR 2
    tablespoons dried parsley flakes
2 tablespoons minced fresh dill weed OR 2 teaspoons
    dried dill

*C*ombine the flour, sugar, and baking powder in a bowl. Stir to mix. Beat the egg, milk, and oil together. Add to the flour mixture along with the remaining ingredients. Mix just until the batter is blended. Spoon into oiled muffin tins or paper muffin cups. Fill about three-fourths full. Bake in a 400-degree oven for 12 to 15 minutes, or until brown.

ONE MUFFIN
=
113 calories
15 CHO
3 PRO
5 FAT
133 SODIUM
49 POTASSIUM
35 CHOLESTEROL

Exchange Value:
1 Bread Exchange +
1 Fat Exchange

APRICOT MUFFINS

(Makes 8)

½ cup finely snipped dried apricots
⅓ cup unsweetened apple juice
1 cup whole wheat flour
2 teaspoons baking powder
¼ teaspoon baking soda
¼ teaspoon ground cardamom
⅓ cup chopped walnuts
3 tablespoons vegetable oil
1 tablespoon sugar
1 egg

ONE MUFFIN

=

182 calories
22 CHO
4 PRO
10 FAT
97 SODIUM
166 POTASSIUM
34 CHOLESTEROL

Exchange Value:
1 Bread Exchange +
½ Fruit Exchange +
2 Fat Exchanges

Soak the apricots in the apple juice for 10 minutes. Combine the flour, baking powder, baking soda, cardamom, and walnuts in a bowl. Beat together the oil, sugar, and egg. Add the apricots, with the juice, and egg mixture to the flour. Mix just until all the ingredients are blended. Spoon into oiled muffin tins, or paper muffin cups, filling three-fourths full. Bake in a 350-degree oven for 10 to 15 minutes, or until golden brown.

CARROT CAKE MUFFIN TREATS

(Makes 12)

1½ cups whole wheat flour
1 teaspoon baking soda
1 tablespoon baking powder
1 teaspoon ground cinnamon
¼ teaspoon ground nutmeg
¼ teaspoon ground ginger
1 egg
2 tablespoons vegetable oil
¼ cup dark or golden raisins
¼ cup chopped walnuts
⅓ cup lowfat milk
1 8-ounce can unsweetened crushed pineapple
1½ cups grated carrots

ONE MUFFIN
=
127 calories
19 CHO
4 PRO
5 FAT
149 SODIUM
201 POTASSIUM
23 CHOLESTEROL

Exchange Value:
1 Bread Exchange +
1 Fat Exchange

Combine the flour, baking soda, baking powder, cinnamon, nutmeg, and ginger in a bowl. Add the remaining ingredients and stir to blend. Spoon into oiled muffin tins or paper muffin cups. Bake in a 350-degree oven for 20 to 25 minutes.

PUMPKIN–BRAN MUFFINS

(Makes 8)

1 cup flour
½ cup bran
1 tablespoon sugar
2 teaspoons baking powder
½ teaspoon baking soda
½ teaspoon ground cinnamon
2 tablespoons vegetable oil
½ cup cooked or canned pumpkin
1 egg
¾ cup orange juice
⅓ cup dark or golden raisins
1 tablespoon wheat germ

ONE MUFFIN
=
148 calories
25 CHO
3 PRO
4 FAT
123 SODIUM
189 POTASSIUM
34 CHOLESTEROL

Exchange Value:
1 Bread Exchange +
1 Fruit Exchange +
1 Fat Exchange

Combine all the ingredients, *except* the wheat germ, in a mixing bowl. Stir to blend. Spoon into lightly oiled muffin tins. Sprinkle on the wheat germ. Bake in a 400-degree oven for 10 to 15 minutes.

BAKING POWDER BISCUITS

(Makes 12)

2 cups flour
3 teaspoons baking powder
¼ teaspoon salt
¼ cup margarine
½ cup lowfat milk

ONE BISCUIT
=
109 calories
15 CHO
2 PRO
4 FAT
152 SODIUM
37 POTASSIUM
0 CHOLESTEROL

Exchange Value:
1 Bread Exchange +
1 Fat Exchange

Combine the flour, baking powder, and salt in a mixing bowl. Cut in the margarine with a fork or pastry blender. Add the milk. Stir to make a soft dough. Roll out on a lightly floured surface until ½ inch thick. Cut into biscuit shapes. Place on an ungreased baking sheet. Bake in a 425-degree oven for 12 to 15 minutes.

LOW-CHOLESTEROL POPOVERS

(Makes 9)

1 cup unbleached white flour
¼ teaspoon salt
1 cup skim milk
1 egg
1 egg white

*P*reheat the oven to 425 degrees. Oil muffin or popover tins and preheat. Combine all the ingredients in a bowl. Beat with a rotary beater or wire whisk just until smooth. Pour the batter into the hot muffin tins. Bake for 35 to 45 minutes, or until brown.

ONE POPOVER
=
68 calories
11 CHO
3 PRO
1 FAT
82 SODIUM
67 POTASSIUM
32 CHOLESTEROL

Exchange Value:
1 Bread Exchange

PUMPKIN PANCAKES

(Makes twenty-four 4-inch pancakes)

1 egg
1 cup milk
½ cup cooked or canned pumpkin
¾ cup unbleached enriched white flour
¾ cup whole wheat flour
2 teaspoons baking powder
1 tablespoon sugar
¼ teaspoon ground cinnamon
⅛ teaspoon ground nutmeg
⅛ teaspoon ground ginger
2 tablespoons vegetable oil

*C*ombine all the ingredients in a mixing bowl and stir just until blended. Pour the batter onto a hot griddle that has been lightly oiled. Flip the pancakes over when bubbles break around edges. Serve hot with rum-flavored fruit sauce.

ONE PANCAKE
=
98 calories
15 CHO
3 PRO
3 FAT
58 SODIUM
96 POTASSIUM
24 CHOLESTEROL

Exchange Value:
1 Bread Exchange +
½ Fat Exchange

WHOLE WHEAT–BUTTERMILK PANCAKES

(Makes twelve 4-inch pancakes)

½ cup whole wheat flour
½ cup unbleached white flour
1 teaspoon sugar
1 teaspoon baking powder
½ teaspoon baking soda
¼ teaspoon salt
1 egg
1 cup buttermilk OR sour milk (1 cup lowfat milk plus
   1 tablespoon vinegar)
2 teaspoons vegetable oil

TWO PANCAKES
=
114 calories
18 CHO
4 PRO
3 FAT
246 SODIUM
1200 POTASSIUM
47 CHOLESTEROL

Exchange Value:
1 Bread Exchange +
½ Fat Exchange

S tir together the flours, sugar, baking powder, baking soda, and salt. Beat the egg, milk, and oil together. Add the liquids to the flour mixture and stir just until blended. Pour the batter onto a greased hot griddle. Serve with fresh fruit slices, unsweetened applesauce, or low-calorie syrup.

CORN BREAD

(Serves 12)

2 cups cornmeal
½ teaspoon salt
½ teaspoon baking soda
2 teaspoons baking powder
1 tablespoon sugar or honey
1 egg
1 tablespoon vegetable oil
1 cup buttermilk OR sour milk (1 cup lowfat milk plus
　1 tablespoon vinegar)

Combine the cornmeal, salt, baking soda, and baking powder in a bowl. Mix to blend. Add the sugar, egg, oil, and milk. Mix well. Pour into a lightly oiled 8-inch-square baking pan. Bake in a 400-degree oven for 20 to 25 minutes.

ONE SERVING
=
113 calories
20 CHO
3 PRO
2 FAT
184 SODIUM
65 POTASSIUM
24 CHOLESTEROL

Exchange Value:
1 Bread Exchange

BANANA BREAD
(Serves 15)

2 cups whole wheat flour
2 teaspoons baking powder
½ teaspoon baking soda
½ teaspoon ground nutmeg
2 eggs
½ cup vegetable oil
2 tablespoons sugar
1½ cups sliced bananas (2 large)

Combine the flour, baking powder, baking soda, and nutmeg in a mixing bowl. Stir to blend. Put the eggs, oil, sugar, and bananas in a blender. Purée until smooth. Pour the banana mixture into the flour. Mix well. Pour into an oiled 9- by 5-inch loaf pan. Bake in a 350-degree oven for 40 to 50 minutes. Cool on a wire rack. Let stand 10 minutes before removing from pan. Cool thoroughly before serving.

**ONE
SERVING**
=
164 calories
21 CHO
3 PRO
8 FAT
70 SODIUM
114 POTASSIUM
37 CHOLESTEROL

Exchange Value:
1 Bread Exchange +
½ Fruit Exchange +
1½ Fat Exchanges

PUMPKIN–RAISIN BREAD

(Serves 15)

⅓ cup vegetable oil
2 tablespoons sugar
2 eggs
¾ cup cooked or canned pumpkin
1 cup unbleached enriched white flour
1 cup whole wheat flour
1 tablespoon baking powder
½ teaspoon baking soda
¼ teaspoon salt
1 teaspoon ground cinnamon
½ cup dark or golden raisins
¼ cup lowfat milk or orange juice

ONE SERVING
=
153 calories
23 CHO
3 PRO
6 FAT
122 SODIUM
117 POTASSIUM
37 CHOLESTEROL

Exchange Value:
1 Bread Exchange +
½ Fruit Exchange +
1 Fat Exchange

*B*eat together the oil, sugar, eggs, and pumpkin until light and fluffy. Combine the flours, baking powder, baking soda, salt, cinnamon, and raisins in a bowl. Stir into the creamed mixture with the milk (or orange juice). Pour into an oiled 9- by 5-inch loaf pan. Bake in a 350-degree oven for 40 to 45 minutes.

CRANBERRY–NUT BREAD

(Serves 15)

1 cup whole wheat flour
1 cup unbleached all-purpose flour
¼ cup sugar
1 tablespoon baking powder
2 teaspoons grated orange rind
1 cup orange juice
2 tablespoons vegetable oil
1 egg
1 cup chopped fresh or frozen cranberries
⅓ cup dark or golden raisins
⅓ cup chopped walnuts

*C*ombine the flours, sugar, baking powder, and orange rind in a mixing bowl. Add the remaining ingredients and stir to blend well. Pour into an oiled 9-by 5-inch loaf pan. Bake in a 350-degree oven for 45 to 50 minutes. Cool for 6 minutes before removing from the pan. Cool thoroughly on a wire rack. Store in a plastic bag or aluminum foil for at least one day before slicing.

ONE SERVING
=

142 calories
24 CHO
3 PRO
4 FAT
55 SODIUM
120 POTASSIUM
18 CHOLESTEROL

Exchange Value:
1 Bread Exchange +
½ Fruit Exchange +
1 Fat Exchange

RUM-FLAVORED FRUIT SAUCE

(Makes 2 cups)

¼ cup boiling water
¼ cup dark or golden raisins
4 ripe bananas, peeled
1 orange, peeled
Juice of 1 lemon
½ to 1 teaspoon rum extract

*P*our the boiling water over the raisins and let stand until the raisins are plump. Then combine all the ingredients in a blender and purée until smooth.
   Delicious on pancakes, waffles, and French toast.

ONE SERVING OF ¼ CUP

=

74 calories
19 CHO
1 PRO
0 FAT
1 SODIUM
289 POTASSIUM
0 CHOLESTEROL

Exchange Value:
1 Fruit Exchange

FRUIT SAUCE FOR PANCAKES

(Makes 1½ cups)

¼ cup boiling water
¼ cup dark or golden raisins
4 ripe bananas, peeled
1 orange, peeled
2 tablespoons lemon juice

*P*our the boiling water over the raisins and let stand until the raisins are plump. Combine all the ingredients in a blender and purée until smooth.

ONE SERVING OF ¼ CUP

=

99 calories
25 CHO
1 PRO
0 FAT
1 SODIUM
386 POTASSIUM
0 CHOLESTEROL

Exchange Value:
1½ Fruit Exchanges

11
SPECIAL CAKES

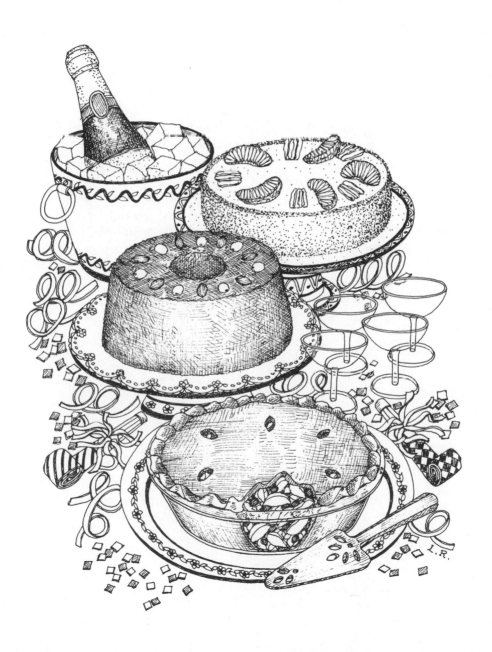

Fruitcakes are holiday traditions in many homes. Dried fruits, such as apricots, prunes, and dates, are better sources of nutrition than the chopped candied fruit that is added to most fruitcake recipes. Orange juice and grated orange rind are used to replace citron in these recipes to give that stimulating contrast of sweet and bitter flavors. Pumpkin is a versatile ingredient that blends well in fruitcake.

F R U I T C A K E

(Serves 15)

½ cup snipped dried figs
½ cup chopped dates
½ cup chopped prunes
1 cup crushed pineapple
1 cup dark raisins
2 cups chopped apple OR 1 medium-size apple,
   chopped
½ cup chopped walnuts
½ cup orange juice
2 cups whole wheat flour
½ cup wheat germ, toasted
1 tablespoon baking powder
1 teaspoon baking soda
1 teaspoon ground cinnamon
½ teaspoon ground nutmeg
2 eggs

Combine the figs, dates, prunes, pineapple, raisins, apple, walnuts, and orange juice in a bowl. Add the remaining ingredients and mix well. Pour into a lightly oiled 10-inch tube pan. Bake in a 350-degree oven for 40 to 50 minutes.

ONE SERVING
=
193 calories
37 CHO
5 PRO
4 FAT
117 SODIUM
349 POTASSIUM
37 CHOLESTEROL

Exchange Value:
1 Bread Exchange +
1½ Fruit Exchanges
+ 1 Fat Exchange

PUMPKIN FRUITCAKE

(Serves 16)

½ cup unsweetened apple juice or orange juice
½ cup dark or golden raisins
1 cup chopped dried figs
1 cup canned or cooked pumpkin
2 tablespoons sugar
¼ cup vegetable oil
1½ cups whole wheat flour
1 teaspoon baking soda
1 teaspoon baking powder
1 teaspoon ground cinnamon
½ teaspoon ground nutmeg
¼ teaspoon ground allspice
⅛ teaspoon ground cloves
½ cup chopped walnuts
Grated rind of 1 orange

ONE SERVING
=
160 calories
26 CHO
3 PRO
6 FAT
69 SODIUM
221 POTASSIUM
0 CHOLESTEROL

Exchange Value:
1 Bread Exchange +
1 Fruit Exchange +
1 Fat Exchange

Combine the juice, raisins, and figs in a bowl. Let stand for 1 hour or overnight.

Beat together the pumpkin, sugar, and oil. Stir in the fruit mixture. Add the flour, baking soda, baking powder, and spices. Mix well. Add the walnuts and orange rind. Stir to blend well. Pour the batter into a lightly oiled 8- by 5-inch loaf pan. Bake in a 325-degree oven for 40 to 45 minutes, or until a toothpick inserted into the center comes out clean. Let cool in the pan for 5 minutes. Remove from the pan and cool thoroughly on a wire rack. Wrap in foil and refrigerate until ready to use.

THYME–FIG FRUITCAKE

(Serves 12)

½ cup unsweetened apple juice
½ teaspoon dried thyme
1 cup finely chopped dried figs
1¼ cups flour
¼ cup cornmeal
2 teaspoons baking powder
¼ teaspoon baking soda
6 tablespoons vegetable oil
2 tablespoons sugar
1 egg
¼ cup pine nuts, toasted

ONE SERVING
=
190 calories
27 CHO
3 PRO
8 FAT
66 SODIUM
156 POTASSIUM
23 CHOLESTEROL

Exchange Value:
1 Bread Exchange +
1 Fruit Exchange +
1½ Fat Exchanges

Combine the apple juice, thyme, and figs in a bowl. Set aside for 10 minutes. Stir together the flour, cornmeal, baking powder, and baking soda in a bowl. Beat the oil, sugar, and egg until well blended. Pour the egg mixture into the flour. Add the pine nuts and fig mixture. Beat well. Pour the batter into an oiled and floured 9-inch-round baking pan. Bake in a 350-degree oven for 40 to 50 minutes. Cool for 5 minutes in the pan. Remove from the pan and cool thoroughly.

12
TURKEY RECIPES
FOR LEFTOVERS

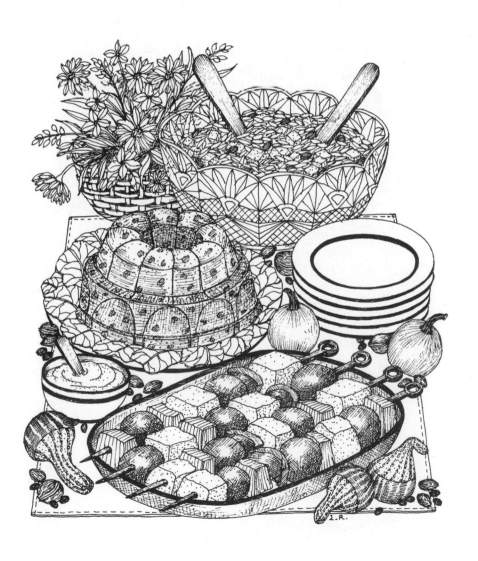

*C*ooking that large turkey for the family holiday meal often leaves leftovers that can be used in tasty meals. Whether you want a salad or a casserole or a soup, you'll find a recipe in this section to whet your appetite.

TACO SALAD WITH CUMIN DRESSING

(Serves 4)

4 tortillas
1 tablespoon grated Parmesan cheese
4 cups Romaine lettuce
¼ teaspoon salt
2 tablespoons red wine vinegar
⅛ teaspoon black pepper
⅛ teaspoon garlic powder
2 teaspoons lemon juice
½ teaspoon powdered mustard
½ teaspoon ground cumin
¼ cup water
2 tablespoons vegetable oil
2 cups chopped cooked turkey
½ teaspoon cumin seeds
3 large ripe tomatoes, chopped
1 cup grated Cheddar cheese

ONE SERVING
=

411 calories
20 CHO
33 PRO
23 FAT
870 SODIUM
617 POTASSIUM
88 CHOLESTEROL

Exchange Value:
4 Lean Meat
Exchanges + 1
Bread Exchange + 1
Vegetable Exchange
+ 2 Fat Exchanges

*T*oast the tortillas on a baking sheet in a 400-degree oven for about 10 minutes. While hot, sprinkle on the Parmesan cheese. Cool and break into bite-size pieces.

Chop the lettuce and arrange it in the bottom of a salad bowl. Make the cumin dressing by combining the salt, vinegar, pepper, garlic powder, lemon juice, mustard, cumin, water, and oil in a bowl or jar. Heat the turkey in a skillet with the cumin seeds. Sprinkle chunks of turkey over the lettuce. Add the tomato pieces and cheese. Pour on the cumin dressing and top with tortilla chips.

SHEPHERD'S TURKEY PIE

(Serves 6)

2 onions, sliced
2 tablespoons vegetable oil
4 cups chopped cooked turkey or chicken
¼ cup whole wheat flour
2 cups chicken stock or broth
2 cups sliced steamed carrots
2 cups diced ripe tomatoes or canned peeled tomatoes
½ teaspoon dried thyme
½ teaspoon dried rosemary
6 potatoes, cooked and mashed

*I*n a large saucepan, sauté the onions in the oil for 5 minutes. Add the turkey (or chicken). Sprinkle in the flour. Stir to blend. Add the chicken stock, carrots, tomatoes, thyme, and rosemary. Cook over medium heat until thickened. Pour into a lightly oiled 3-quart casserole. Spread the potatoes over the top. Bake in a 375-degree oven for 20 to 30 minutes, or until browned.

ONE SERVING
=
371 calories
38 CHO
33 PRO
10 FAT
81 SODIUM
1133 POTASSIUM
71 CHOLESTEROL

Exchange Value:
4 Lean Meat
Exchanges + 2
Bread Exchanges +
1 Vegetable Exchange

CURRIED TURKEY ON RICE

(Serves 4)

1 apple, chopped
1 onion, chopped
3 tablespoons margarine
¼ cup flour
½ teaspoon salt
2 to 3 teaspoons curry powder
1 cup lowfat milk
2 cups diced cooked turkey
Cooked brown rice

Sauté the apple and onion in the margarine until the onion is tender. Stir in the flour, salt, and curry powder. Slowly add the milk. Cook, stirring constantly, until thickened. Stir in the turkey. Simmer, stirring occasionally, until hot and bubbly. Serve on the rice.

ONE SERVING
=
353 calories
32 CHO
26 PRO
13 FAT
306 SODIUM
408 POTASSIUM
56 CHOLESTEROL

Exchange Value:
3 Lean Meat
Exchanges + 2
Bread Exchanges +
1 Fat Exchange

TURKEY–ORANGE SALAD

(Serves 4)

2 cups chopped cooked turkey
½ cup chopped celery
¼ teaspoon salt
¼ teaspoon curry powder
1 orange
1 cup seedless grapes
2 tablespoons mayonnaise or salad dressing
1 tablespoon shredded coconut, toasted

Combine the turkey, celery, salt, and curry powder in a bowl. Peel and chop the orange. Add the orange, grapes, and mayonnaise to the turkey. Toss gently to mix. Sprinkle on the coconut just before serving.

ONE SERVING
=

217 calories
12 CHO
21 PRO
10 FAT
228 SODIUM
391 POTASSIUM
58 CHOLESTEROL

Exchange Value:
3 Lean Meat Exchanges + 1 Fruit Exchange

CURRY TURKEY STIR-FRY

(Serves 4)

2 cups chopped cooked turkey
1½ to 2 teaspoons curry powder
1 tablespoon soy sauce
4 green onions (scallions), chopped
4 celery stalks, chopped thin
1 pound fresh pea pods, snipped
1 sweet red pepper, sliced
1 tablespoon cornstarch
1½ cups water

Heat a nonstick wok or skillet. Add the turkey, curry powder, soy sauce, and onions. Sauté until the turkey is heated, about 2 minutes. Add the celery, pea pods, and pepper. Stir-fry another 3 to 4 minutes. Add the cornstarch that has been dissolved in the water. Cook just until the liquid thickens.

ONE SERVING
=

151 calories
7 CHO
22 PRO
4 FAT
285 SODIUM
404 POTASSIUM
54 CHOLESTEROL

Exchange Value:
3 Lean Meat Exchanges + 1 Vegetable Exchange

WILD RICE–TURKEY SALAD

(Serves 4)

½ cup wild rice
1½ cups water
2 cups chopped cooked turkey
1 cup chopped celery
½ cup chopped sweet red pepper (optional)
⅓ cup golden raisins
1 apple, chopped
¼ cup chopped green onions (scallions)
¼ cup olive oil
2 tablespoons red or white wine vinegar
¼ teaspoon black pepper
¼ teaspoon ground nutmeg
2 tablespoons chopped fresh parsley leaves
Chopped pecans for garnish

Cook the rice in the water until tender, about 50 minutes. Cut the turkey into bite-size pieces. Combine all the ingredients in a bowl and toss. Cover and chill until ready to serve. Sprinkle on the pecans just before serving.

ONE SERVING
=

422 calories
43 CHO
24 PRO
18 FAT
344 SODIUM
503 POTASSIUM
54 CHOLESTEROL

Exchange Value:
3 Lean Meat Exchanges + 1 Bread Exchange + 1½ Fruit Exchanges + 1 Vegetable Exchange + 2 Fat Exchanges

HAWAIIAN
TURKEY KEBOBS
(Serves 4)

1 pound cooked turkey, cut into 1-inch cubes
1 8-ounce can juice-packed pineapple chunks
1 medium-size onion, cut into quarters
1 sweet green pepper, cut into squares
10 to 12 cherry tomatoes
1 tablespoon soy sauce
½ teaspoon curry powder
¼ teaspoon ground ginger

*B*egin each skewer with a cube of turkey. Add pineapple. Separate the onion into pieces and add one piece; then add the green pepper and tomato. Repeat. Put the skewers in a baking pan. Combine the soy sauce, pineapple juice, curry powder, and ginger. Pour over the kebobs. Bake in a 400-degree oven for 15 minutes, turning frequently to coat with the sauce. Serve on rice, if desired.

ONE SERVING (rice not included)
=

177 calories
14 CHO
22 PRO
4 FAT
271 SODIUM
453 POTASSIUM
54 CHOLESTEROL

Exchange Value:
3 Lean Meat Exchanges + ½ Fruit Exchange + 1 Vegetable Exchange

TURKEY GUMBO

(Serves 4)

2 tablespoons margarine
½ pound fresh or frozen okra, cut into 1-inch lengths
2 cups chopped celery
1 medium-size onion, chopped
1 small sweet green pepper, chopped
2 garlic cloves, minced
1 8-ounce can tomato paste
4 ripe tomatoes, peeled, OR 1 16-ounce can peeled
  tomatoes
2 cups water
2 cups chopped cooked turkey
¾ teaspoon gumbo file powder
Cooked rice

M elt the margarine in a large skillet. Add the okra.
Sauté until the okra loses its shiny appearance, about 5
minutes. Remove the okra pieces to a bowl. Add the
celery, onion, green pepper, and garlic to the skillet.
Cook over medium heat until the onion is transparent.
Add the tomato paste, tomatoes, water, okra mixture,
and turkey. Cook over low heat 10 minutes or until
turkey is hot. Add the file powder. Stir to blend. Spoon
over the rice in soup bowls.

**ONE
SERVING
(rice not
included)**
=
*255 calories
19 CHO
25 PRO
10 FAT
176 SODIUM
1102 POTASSIUM
54 CHOLESTEROL*

*Exchange Value:
3 Lean Meat
Exchanges + 1
Bread Exchange + 1
Vegetable Exchange*

MOLDED TURKEY–PINEAPPLE SALAD

(Serves 4)

1 tablespoon unflavored gelatin
1¼ cups pineapple juice
¾ cup chicken broth
3 cups chopped cooked turkey
1 8-ounce can crushed pineapple in juice, drained
20 seedless green grapes, cut in half
½ cup finely chopped celery
¼ cup chopped sweet red pepper
2 tablespoons minced green onion (scallion)

Dissolve the gelatin in ¼ cup of the pineapple juice. Let sit for 5 minutes. Boil the chicken broth and pour it over the gelatin. Stir to dissolve. Add the remaining cup of pineapple juice and chill until thickened.

Meanwhile, combine the remaining ingredients in a bowl. Pour the gelatin mixture over the turkey and pour into a 9- by 5-inch loaf pan. Refrigerate overnight or at least 4 hours. Cut into squares and serve on lettuce.

ONE SERVING
=
286 calories
27 CHO
32 PRO
6 FAT
86 SODIUM
594 POTASSIUM
80 CHOLESTEROL

Exchange Value:
4 Lean Meat Exchanges + 1 Vegetable Exchange + 1½ Fruit Exchanges

LOW-CALORIE
TURKEY–SPINACH LASAGNA

(Serves 8)

3 10-ounce boxes frozen chopped spinach
16 ounces lowfat ricotta cheese
2 cups chopped cooked turkey
2 cups OR 1 15-ounce jar spaghetti sauce
8 ounces lowfat mozzarella cheese, sliced
¼ cup grated Parmesan cheese

*T*haw the spinach and squeeze out any liquid. Put about one third of the spinach in the bottom of a lightly oiled casserole. Spread half of the ricotta over the spinach. Sprinkle on half of the turkey. Spoon on half of the spaghetti sauce. Top with half of the mozzarella slices. Repeat the layering process using another third of the spinach; then the rest of the ricotta, turkey, spaghetti sauce, and mozzarella. Finish with the final third of spinach. Sprinkle on the Parmesan cheese. Bake in a 350-degree oven for 45 to 50 minutes, or until browned.

**ONE
SERVING**
=

*260 calories
9 CHO
23 PRO
15 FAT
590 SODIUM
502 POTASSIUM
62 CHOLESTEROL*

*Exchange Value:
3 Lean Meat
Exchanges + 2
Vegetable Exchanges
+ 1 Fat Exchange*

TURKEY CHOWDER

(Serves 6)

½ cup chopped onion
1 cup sliced celery
2 tablespoons margarine
2 tablespoons flour
½ teaspoon salt
¼ teaspoon ground black pepper
1 teaspoon dried thyme
5 cups turkey or chicken broth
2 potatoes, peeled and cubed
1 cup chopped carrots
1 cup sliced zucchini
½ cup unsweetened apple juice
3 cups cooked chopped turkey

ONE SERVING
=
222 calories
16 CHO
23 PRO
8 FAT
282 SODIUM
570 POTASSIUM
54 CHOLESTEROL

Exchange Value:
3 Lean Meat
Exchanges + 1
Bread Exchange

*S*auté the onion and celery in the margarine. Add the flour, salt, pepper, and thyme. Gradually add the broth. Add the potatoes and carrots. Cover and simmer for 15 minutes, or until the vegetables are tender. Add the zucchini, apple juice, and turkey. Continue cooking over low heat for 10 minutes.

TURKEY CHILI
(Serves 4)

2 cups chopped cooked turkey
1 garlic clove, minced
1 medium-size onion, chopped
1 sweet green pepper, chopped
17 ounces red kidney beans, canned
1 6-ounce can tomato paste
1 28-ounce can tomatoes
1 bay leaf
1 to 2 tablespoons chili powder
½ teaspoon cumin seeds

Combine the turkey, garlic, onion, and green pepper in a nonstick skillet. Sauté until the vegetables are soft. Add the remaining ingredients and cover. Simmer over low heat for 30 to 60 minutes, or until the flavors are blended.

ONE SERVING
=
340 calories
33 CHO
30 PRO
10 FAT
355 SODIUM
1211 POTASSIUM
60 CHOLESTEROL

Exchange Value:
3 Lean Meat
Exchanges + 1
Bread Exchange + 2
Vegetable Exchanges

TURKEY–BARLEY SOUP

(Serves 6)

6 cups turkey or chicken broth
1 cup diced cooked turkey
1 cup pearl barley
1 onion, chopped
2 celery stalks, chopped
3 carrots, sliced
1 bay leaf
1 teaspoon dried thyme
¼ teaspoon dried marjoram
¼ teaspoon ground black pepper
2 tablespoons chopped fresh parsley leaves

Combine all the ingredients in soup pot or slow cooker. Cook over low heat in the slow cooker for 6 hours, or simmer on the stove for 1 hour, or until the carrots are tender and the barley is soft.

ONE SERVING
=
181 calories
30 CHO
11 PRO
2 FAT
44 SODIUM
320 POTASSIUM
18 CHOLESTEROL

Exchange Value:
1 Lean Meat
Exchange + 1 Bread
Exchange + 2
Vegetable Exchanges

SPICY RICE PILAF WITH TURKEY

(Serves 4)

1 cup brown rice
½ teaspoon cumin seeds
¼ teaspoon ground ginger
¼ teaspoon ground cinnamon
4 cardamom seeds
4 whole cloves
1 tablespoon vegetable oil
2 cups turkey stock or water
¼ cup dark or golden raisins
2 cups chopped cooked turkey
¼ cup pine nuts or chopped cashews, toasted

*S*auté the rice, cumin seeds, ginger, cinnamon, cardamom seeds, and cloves in the oil in a saucepan until the rice is browned. Add the stock (or water) and bring the mixture to a boil. Lower the heat and simmer for 45 to 50 minutes, or until the rice is cooked. Add the raisins, turkey, and nuts to the rice mixture. Serve hot or cold.

ONE SERVING
=
317 calories
24 CHO
25 PRO
14 FAT
190 SODIUM
381 POTASSIUM
54 CHOLESTEROL

Exchange Value:
3 Lean Meat Exchanges +
1 Bread Exchange +
½ Fruit Exchange +
1 Fat Exchange

TURKEY BARBECUE FOR SANDWICHES

(Serves 4)

1 16-ounce can tomatoes, cut up
1 6-ounce can tomato paste
1 teaspoon powdered mustard
¼ cup chopped onion
1 to 2 teaspoons chili powder
2 cups chopped cooked turkey

Combine all the ingredients in a saucepan. Simmer for 10 to 15 minutes, or until the flavors are blended. Spoon the mixture over hamburger buns.

ONE SERVING (buns not included)
=
176 calories
12 CHO
23 PRO
4 FAT
220 SODIUM
767 POTASSIUM
54 CHOLESTEROL

Exchange Value:
3 Lean Meat Exchanges + 2 Vegetable Exchanges
(buns not included)

TURKEY SPAGHETTI SAUCE

(Serves 6)

¼ cup chopped onion
1 garlic clove, minced
1 teaspoon olive oil
1 28-ounce can tomatoes, cut up
1 6-ounce can tomato paste
1 teaspoon dried basil
1 teaspoon dried thyme
3 cups chopped cooked turkey
Cooked noodles or macaroni

*S*auté the onion and garlic in the oil until lightly browned. Add the tomatoes, tomato paste, basil, thyme, and turkey. Simmer for 20 to 25 minutes while cooking the noodles or macaroni.

ONE SERVING (noodles or macaroni not included)
=
215 calories
9 CHO
22 PRO
10 FAT
190 SODIUM
627 POTASSIUM
54 CHOLESTEROL

Exchange Value:
3 Lean Meat
Exchanges + 2
Vegetable Exchanges
(noodles or macaroni
not included)

TURKEY FRITTATA

(Serves 6)

½ cup sliced onion
1 garlic clove, minced
1 tablespoon oil
1 cup sliced mushrooms
1 cup frozen chopped spinach, defrosted and
   squeezed dry
2 tablespoons lemon juice
⅛ teaspoon ground black pepper
1 cup chopped cooked turkey
6 eggs, beaten

ONE SERVING
=
158 calories
4 CHO
15 PRO
9 FAT
106 SODIUM
318 POTASSIUM
292 CHOLESTEROL

Exchange Value:
2 Lean Meat
Exchanges + 1
Vegetable Exchange
+ ½ Fat Exchange

Sauté the onion, garlic, and mushrooms in the oil for 5 minutes. Add the spinach, lemon juice, and pepper. Cook over low heat for 3 minutes. Add the turkey and eggs to the spinach mixture. Pour into a greased 9-inch-round baking pan. Bake in a 350-degree oven for 25 to 30 minutes, or until the eggs are set. Cut into wedges to serve.

13

TRADITIONAL JEWISH RECIPES

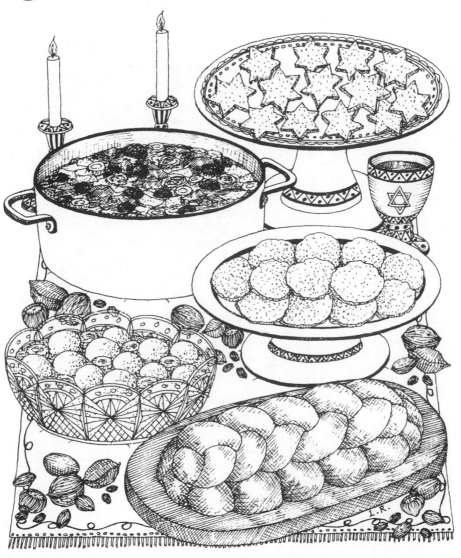

J ewish dietary principles restrict certain combinations of foods at meals and in recipes. These recipes have been modified to meet those dietary restrictions and provide lowfat, low-salt, and low-sugar foods.

BEEF CHOLENT
(Sabbath Meal-in-One)

(Serves 6)

1½ pounds lean beef pot roast
1 onion, chopped
1 cup lima beans, soaked overnight in water to cover
2 potatoes, peeled and cut into quarters
4 carrots, cut into 1-inch chunks
½ teaspoon salt
½ teaspoon ground black pepper
2 bay leaves

Brown the pot roast in a nonstick pan with the onion. Combine with the remaining ingredients in a Dutch oven or crock pot. Add enough water to cover the ingredients. Cover tightly and simmer slowly in a 200-degree oven or crock pot overnight.

ONE SERVING
=
386 calories
33 CHO
39 PRO
11 FAT
253 SODIUM
1223 POTASSIUM
72 CHOLESTEROL

Exchange Values:
4 Medium-Fat Meat Exchanges + 2 Bread Exchanges

L A T K E S
(Potato Pancakes)

(Serves 4)

2 large baking potatoes
1 tablespoon grated onion
1 egg
⅓ cup flour
1 cup vegetable oil
Plain lowfat yogurt
Unsweetened applesauce

*P*eel and grate the potatoes onto paper towels. Squeeze out the moisture. Combine the potatoes and the remaining ingredients *except* the yogurt and applesauce. Beat well. Heat the oil in a skillet. Drop the batter into the oil by spoonfuls. Fry until crisp and brown on both sides. Remove from the skillet and drain on paper towels. Serve warm with plain yogurt and unsweetened applesauce.

Note: One-fourth cup oil is used in frying. Reserve rest of oil for later use by storing in the refrigerator.

ONE SERVING of 3 pancakes (yogurt and applesauce not included)
=
260 calories
27 CHO
5 PRO
15 FAT
23 SODIUM
449 POTASSIUM
66 CHOLESTEROL

Exchange Values:
2 Bread Exchanges
+ 3 Fat Exchanges
(yogurt and applesauce not included)

ZIMSTERNE
(Spicy Star Cookies)
(Makes 60)

¼ cup margarine
¼ cup honey
¼ cup sugar
2 eggs
3 cups flour
2 teaspoons baking powder
½ teaspoon baking soda
1 teaspoon ground cinnamon
½ teaspoon ground nutmeg
¼ teaspoon ground cloves
½ cup unsweetened apple juice

ONE SERVING of 2 cookies

=

78 calories
14 CHO
2 PRO
2 FAT
52 SODIUM
22 POTASSIUM
9 CHOLESTEROL

Exchange Value:
1 Bread Exchange

Cream the margarine, honey, sugar, and eggs together in a bowl until smooth and fluffy. Add the remaining ingredients and mix well. Divide the dough into thirds. Flatten each one into a circle ½ inch thick. Wrap each in plastic wrap. Refrigerate overnight until firm.

   Remove the dough from the refrigerator and roll out on a lightly floured surface to ⅛ inch thick. Cut out the dough with a star cookie cutter and place on a lightly oiled baking sheet. Bake in a 375-degree oven for 8 to 10 minutes, or until lightly browned.

Note: These Zimsterne have approximately three-quarters teaspoon of sugar per serving.

LAMB AND
BROWN RICE PILAF
(Serves 4)

1 large onion, chopped fine
2 garlic cloves, minced
2 celery stalks, chopped fine
1 tablespoon vegetable oil
1 cup brown rice
1 pound boneless lamb, cut into ½-inch cubes
3 cups water
1 15-ounce can garbanzo beans (chick-peas), drained
½ cup dark raisins
1 apple, peeled, cored, and chopped
½ cup finely chopped fresh parsley leaves
½ teaspoon ground allspice
¼ teaspoon ground cinnamon
½ teaspoon dried thyme
¼ teaspoon ground black pepper

**ONE
SERVING**
=
*318 calories
41 CHO
22 PRO
8 FAT
238 SODIUM
518 POTASSIUM
70 CHOLESTEROL*

*Exchange Value:
3 Lean Meat
Exchanges +
2 Bread Exchanges
+ 1 Fruit Exchange*

Sauté the onion, garlic, and celery in the oil in a large pot until tender. Add the rice and cook for 1 minute. Add the lamb cubes and stir to brown on all sides. Add the remaining ingredients and bring to a boil. Lower the heat, cover, and simmer for 45 minutes, or until the rice is tender. Toss with a fork just before serving.

GEFILTE FISH

(Serves 18)

1 pound fresh or frozen whitefish or turbot fillets
1 pound fresh or frozen pike fillets
2 onions, sliced
4 cups water
2 carrots, sliced
1 teaspoon salt
½ teaspoon ground white pepper
2 eggs
¼ cup matzo meal

Defrost the fish, if frozen. Save the head, skin, and bones of fish when filleting. Place them in a large saucepan with the onions, water, carrots, salt, and pepper. Cook over high heat until the fish is ready.

Grind the fish in a food processor. Add the eggs and matzo meal. Mix until well blended. Drop balls of the fish mixture into the fish stock. Cover and simmer for 30 minutes. Remove the cover and continue cooking for 10 minutes longer. Cool the fish balls and place on a platter or in a bowl. Strain the fish stock over fish balls. Add the carrots around the fish. Chill. Serve with horseradish.

ONE SERVING of 2 fish balls
=

98 calories
2 CHO
12 PRO
4 FAT
190 SODIUM
290 POTASSIUM
56 CHOLESTEROL

Exchange Value:
2 Lean Meat
Exchanges

*T*ZIMMES
(Main-Dish Meat and Vegetables)
(Serves 6)

3 carrots
2 potatoes, peeled
1 sweet potato, peeled
1½ pounds beef top round steak
1 onion, sliced thin
½ cup dried prunes
½ cup dried apricots
1 cup orange juice
Water

*C*ut the vegetables into 1-inch pieces. Cut the beef into strips. Brown the meat in a nonstick pan. Add the vegetables, prunes, apricots, and orange juice. Add enough water to cover meat and vegetables. Bring to a boil, lower the heat, and simmer for 2 to 3 hours, or until the meat is tender. Or bake in a 350-degree oven for 3 hours in a covered dish.

ONE SERVING
=
356 calories
41 CHO
35 PRO
7 FAT
100 SODIUM
1113 POTASSIUM
70 CHOLESTEROL

Exchange Value:
4 Lean Meat Exchanges +
1½ Bread Exchanges + 2 Fruit Exchanges

BAKED GEFILTE FISH

(Serves 6)

1 pound fresh or frozen halibut or turbot fillets
1 small onion
1 slice bread, crumbled
½ teaspoon salt
¼ teaspoon ground black pepper
1 egg
1 tablespoon vegetable oil
1 onion, sliced
1 sweet green pepper, chopped
1 8-ounce can tomato sauce

ONE SERVING of 2 fish balls
=
189 calories
9 CHO
20 PRO
8 FAT
671 SODIUM
606 POTASSIUM
77 CHOLESTEROL

Exchange Value:
3 Lean Meat
Exchanges + 1
Vegetable Exchange

*D*efrost the fish, if frozen. Grind the fish and onion in a food processor. Add the bread, salt, pepper, and egg. Mix well. Shape into 12 balls. Combine the oil, onion, green pepper, and tomato sauce in a baking dish. Arrange the fish balls in it, cover, and bake in a 325-degree oven for 40 to 45 minutes. Baste with the sauce before serving.

M A N D E L B R O T
(Almond Bread)
(Serves 18)

3 eggs
⅓ cup sugar
2 tablespoons vegetable oil
1 teaspoon vanilla extract
1¼ cups flour
1 teaspoon baking powder
⅓ cup chopped blanched almonds
2 teaspoons ground cinnamon

*B*eat the eggs and sugar together until thick. Add the oil and vanilla and mix well. Stir in the flour, baking powder, and almonds. Pour the batter into a lightly oiled and floured 9- by 5- by 3-inch loaf pan just to cover the bottom of the pan. Sprinkle on the cinnamon. Add another layer of batter and cinnamon. Continue until all the batter and cinnamon are used. Bake in a 350-degree oven for 20 to 25 minutes, or until golden brown. Bread will be dense. Remove from the pan and cool on a wire rack. Cut into ½-inch slices when ready to serve. Place each slice on a lightly oiled baking sheet and toast in a 400-degree oven for 5 to 6 minutes.

Note: The Mandelbrot has about three-quarters teaspoons of sugar per serving.

**ONE
SERVING**
=
55 calories
6 CHO
1 PRO
3 FAT
13 SODIUM
11 POTASSIUM
44 CHOLESTEROL

Exchange Value:
½ Fruit Exchange +
½ Fat Exchange

CHALLAH
(Holiday Twist Bread)

(Serves 18)

1 package (or 1 tablespoon) active dry yeast
2 tablespoons sugar
¼ cup warm water (110 to 115 degrees)
2 cups all-purpose flour
2 to 2½ cups whole wheat flour
½ teaspoon salt
1 egg
2 tablespoons vegetable oil
1¼ cups water
Beaten egg
1 tablespoon poppy seeds

ONE SERVING
=
115 calories
21 CHO
4 PRO
2 FAT
59 SODIUM
74 POTASSIUM
15 CHOLESTEROL

Exchange Value:
1½ Bread Exchanges

Dissolve the yeast and sugar in the ¼ cup of warm water. Let stand for 5 minutes. Combine the flours and salt in a mixing bowl. Make a well in the center of the flour mixture and add the egg, oil, yeast mixture, and remaining 1¼ cups of water. Mix well. Knead the dough on a floured board, adding more whole wheat flour until the dough is smooth and elastic. Place in an oiled bowl. Cover with a damp towel and let rise until doubled, about 1 hour.

Divide the dough into three parts. Roll each third into a strip about 15 inches long. Braid the strips together and place on a lightly oiled baking sheet. Brush with the beaten egg. Sprinkle on the poppy seeds. Cover and let rise until doubled. Bake in a 375-degree oven for 40 to 45 minutes, or until golden brown.

H O N E Y C A K E

(Serves 24)

3 eggs
¼ cup sugar
¼ cup soft margarine
2½ cups flour
1 teaspoon baking powder
1 teaspoon baking soda
½ teaspoon ground cinnamon
¼ teaspoon ground nutmeg
⅛ teaspoon ground cloves
¼ cup honey
1 cup cold strong coffee
1 ripe banana, mashed

**ONE
SERVING**
=
93 calories
15 CHO
2 PRO
3 FAT
76 SODIUM
41 POTASSIUM
33 CHOLESTEROL

Exchange Value:
1 Bread Exchange +
½ Fat Exchange

*B*eat the eggs until thick. Add the sugar gradually. Beat in the margarine. Stir the flour, baking powder, baking soda, cinnamon, nutmeg, and cloves together. Add gradually to the creamed mixture with the honey and coffee. Beat until combined. Add the banana. Pour the batter into a lightly oiled and floured 10-inch tube pan or two 9-inch loaf pans. Bake in a 350-degree oven for 45 to 50 minutes. Remove from the oven and cool on a wire rack for 5 minutes before removing from the pan. Cool thoroughly before slicing.

Note: The Honey Cake has 1 teaspoon of sugar per serving.

KAESE BLINTZES
(Rolled Cheese Pancakes)
(Serves 6)

1 cup dry cottage cheese
1 cup pot cheese or lowfat ricotta cheese
1 egg
1 tablespoon sugar
1 cup flour
1 cup lowfat milk
3 eggs
Vegetable oil
2 tablespoons margarine
Plain lowfat yogurt

*M*ake the cheese filling by beating cottage cheese, pot cheese, 1 egg, and sugar together. Combine the flour and milk with the 3 eggs. Beat to make a smooth batter.

Heat a 6- or 8-inch skillet. Coat with vegetable oil and pour in 2 to 3 tablespoons of the batter. Tilt the pan to distribute the batter over the bottom of the skillet. Cook until the dough is firm and browned. Remove from the pan and place on a lightly oiled plate with browned side up. Spoon 1 tablespoon of filling onto the edge of the pancake. Roll up by bringing the edge with the filling to the center of the pancake, fold in each side, and fold over once more to make a sealed pouch. Continue with the rest of the batter. When ready to serve, heat the margarine in a skillet. Fry the blintzes until golden brown on all sides. Serve with yogurt.

**ONE
SERVING of 2
blintzes**
=
*272 calories
20 CHO
16 PRO
14 FAT
150 SODIUM
178 POTASSIUM
193 CHOLESTEROL*

*Exchange Value:
2 Lean Meat Exchanges
+ 1 Bread Exchange +
2 Fat Exchanges*

LOKSHEN KUGEL
(Noodle Pudding)
(Serves 6)

2 eggs
1 tablespoon sugar
¼ teaspoon ground nutmeg
2½ cups cooked broad noodles
1 tablespoon vegetable oil
1 cup unsweetened apple juice
½ cup dark or golden raisins
¼ cup chopped walnuts or pecans

*B*eat the eggs and sugar until fluffy. Add the remaining ingredients, *except* the nuts. Pour into a well-oiled 2-quart casserole dish or an 8-inch baking pan. Sprinkle on the nuts. Bake in a 350-degree oven for 40 to 50 minutes, or until browned.

ONE SERVING
=
225 calories
33 CHO
6 PRO
8 FAT
27 SODIUM
215 POTASSIUM
88 CHOLESTEROL

Exchange Value:
1½ Bread Exchanges + 1½ Fruit Exchanges + 1½ Fat Exchanges

MEATY SPLIT PEA SOUP
(Serves 4)

4 cups water
1 cup split peas, sorted and washed
½ pound beef flank steak
½ teaspoon salt
¼ teaspoon ground black pepper
2 carrots, grated
2 onions, chopped

*C*ombine the water and peas in a saucepan. Bring to a boil; then cook over low heat for 1 hour. Cut the beef diagonally into thin slices. Add the beef and the remaining ingredients. Cover and simmer for about 30 minutes, or until the meat is tender. Remove the beef slices and purée if a smooth soup is desired. Serve with the beef slices on top.

ONE SERVING
=
218 calories
27 CHO
23 PRO
3 FAT
298 SODIUM
595 POTASSIUM
35 CHOLESTEROL

Exchange Value:
3 Lean Meat Exchanges + 1 Bread Exchange + 1 Vegetable Exchange

SWEET AND SOUR GREEN BEANS

(Serves 4)

1 10-ounce package frozen green beans
½ cup water
1 bay leaf
4 whole cloves
2 tablespoons red or white wine vinegar
1 tablespoon margarine
1 package Equal sweetener

Combine the beans, water, bay leaf, and cloves in a saucepan. Cook until the beans are tender, about 3 minutes. Drain off the water. Add the vinegar and margarine. Sauté for 3 minutes. Remove the bay leaf and cloves. Sprinkle on the sweetener and serve.

ONE SERVING
=
46 calories
0 CHO
1 PRO
3 FAT
37 SODIUM
39 POTASSIUM
0 CHOLESTEROL

Exchange Value:
1 Vegetable Exchange
+ ½ Fat Exchange

14

MEAL PLANNING
AND
FOOD EXCHANGES

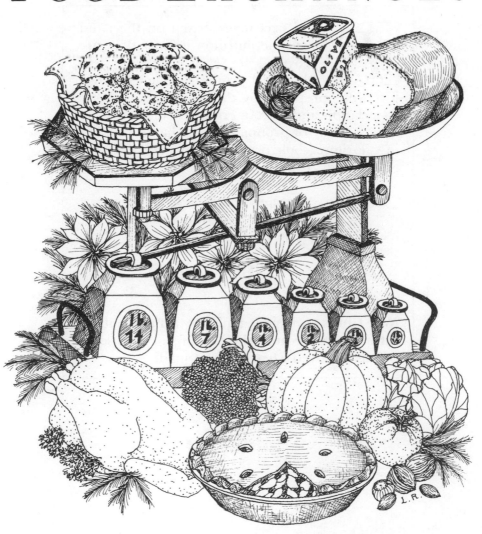

Food exchanges, based on the latest available nutrition information, are provided for each recipe to help with meal planning. The exchange lists were prepared by the American Diabetes Association and the American Dietetic Association as a way of grouping foods that are similar in calorie, carbohydrate, protein, and fat content. These groups of foods are:

Starches and Breads
Meat and Substitutes
Vegetables
Fruits
Milk
Fat

Note: Cheese is included in the **Meat and Substitutes** group because the "sugar" or lactose in milk is removed when cheese is made.

How to Use the Food Exchanges

H ere is how the food exchanges are used with the Thanksgiving Dinner menu given in chapter 3.

Spicy Tomato Cocktail
Potato Hors d'Oeuvres   Salmon Dip
Roast Turkey and Apricot Dressing
Cranapple Relish
Brussels Sprouts with Walnuts   Sweet Potatoes à l'Orange
Traditional Waldorf Salad
Pumpkin–Bran Muffins   Banana Bread
Beverage

Menu Item	Food Exchange	Calories per Serving
Spicy Tomato Cocktail	2 Vegetables	38
Potato Hors d'Oeuvres	1 Bread	50
Salmon Dip	FREE	17
Roast Turkey	3 Lean Meats	175
Apricot Dressing	1 Bread, ½ Fat, ½ Fruit	118
Cranapple Relish	½ Fruit	39
Brussels Sprouts with Walnuts	1 Vegetable, 1½ Fats	100
Sweet Potatoes à l'Orange	1 Bread, 1 Fruit, 1 Fat	185
Traditional Waldorf Salad	2 Fruits, 1½ Fats	147
Pumpkin–Bran Muffins	1 Bread, 1 Fruit, 1 Fat	148
Banana Bread	1 Bread, ½ Fruit, 1½ Fats	164

The meal plan of a person on a 2200-calorie diabetic diet might include these food exchanges for the Thanksgiving Dinner:

3 Lean Meats
3 Starches/Breads
2 Vegetables
2 Fruits
1 Milk
3 Fats

Now the deciding begins. How do you choose what to eat with all these goodies available? Here are some ways to enjoy your Thanksgiving Dinner and still live within the food exchange plan allowed. Of course, the options given are only examples and are designed to teach you how varied your menu can be.

Option 1:	Salmon Dip with 4 Celery Sticks	FREE
	1 Potato Hors d'Oeuvre	1 Bread
	3 ounces Roast Turkey	3 Lean Meats
	Sweet Potatoes à l'Orange	1 Bread, 1 Fruit, 1 Fat
	Brussels Sprouts with Walnuts	1 Vegetable, 1½ Fats
	Pumpkin–Bran Muffin	1 Bread, 1 Fruit, 1 Fat
	8-ounce glass Skim Milk	1 Milk

3 Lean Meats
3 Bread
1 Vegetable
2 Fruits
1 Milk
3½ Fats

Option 2: Instead of having the milk exchange, an extra bread or starch will be selected. This person hates Brussels sprouts!

	Spicy Tomato Cocktail	2 Vegetables
	2 Potato Hors d'Oeuvres	2 Breads
	3 ounces Roast Turkey	3 Lean Meats
	Apricot Dressing (½ serving)	½ Bread, ¼ Fat, ¼ Fruit
	Cranapple Relish (½ serving)	¼ Fruit
	Sweet Potatoes à l'Orange	1 Bread, 1 Fruit, 1 Fat
	Banana Bread	1 Bread, ½ Fruit, 1½ Fats

3 Lean Meats
4½ Breads
2 Vegetables
2 Fruits
0 Milk (added 1 Bread)
2¾ Fats

   Of course, it is easier for the person on 2200 calories to choose from such a selection of holiday foods and still stay within his food exchange plan. When calories are limited, it becomes *much* more difficult to show the restraint needed. Here is how a person on a 1200-calorie diabetic diet might include these exchanges in his Thanksgiving Dinner. The meal plan is:

3 Lean Meats
2 Starches/Breads
2 Vegetables
1 Fruit
2 Fats

Option 1:   Salmon Dip with 4 celery sticks   FREE
               1 Potato Hors d'Oeuvre   1 Bread
               3 ounces Roast Turkey   3 Lean Meats
               Brussels Sprouts with Walnuts   1 Vegetable, 1½ Fats
               Pumpkin–Bran Muffin   <u>1 Bread, 1 Fruit, 1 Fat</u>

                                                    3 Lean Meats
                                                    2 Breads
                                                    1 Vegetable
                                                    1 Fruit
                                                    2½ Fats

Option 2:   This person is the one who likes to sample a little bit of everything. That way he really feels like it was a "holiday" celebration.

               Spicy Tomato Cocktail (½ portion)   1 Vegetable
               1 Potato Hors d'Oeuvre   1 Bread
                3 ounces Roast Turkey   3 Lean Meats
               Apricot Dressing (½ serving)   ½ Bread, ¼ Fat, ¼ Fruit
               Cranapple Relish   ½ Fruit
               Brussels Sprouts with Walnuts   ½ Vegetable, ¾ Fat
                 (½ serving)
               Traditional Waldorf Salad (½ serving)   1 Fruit, ¾ Fat
               Banana Bread (½ slice)   <u>½ Bread, ¼ Fruit, ¾ Fat</u>

                                                      3 Lean Meats
                                                      2 Breads
                                                    1½ Vegetables
                                                      2 Fruits
                                                    2½ Fats

    Exchange lists allow people to choose a wide variety of foods from different food groups without having to count calories or consult a nutrition table for the carbohydrate, protein, and fat content of each food eaten. One food within an exchange list can be substituted or traded for another food in the same list. Be sure to use the portion sizes as stated to keep the carbohydrate, protein, and fat content the same.

Starch/Bread List

Each item in this list contains about 15 grams of carbohydrate, 3 grams of protein, a trace of fat, and 80 calories.

Whole grain products average about 2 grams of fiber per serving. Some foods are higher in fiber.

You can choose your starch servings from any of the items on this list. If you want to eat a starch food that is not on this list, the general rule is:

- ½ cup of cereal, grain, or pasta is one serving
- 1 ounce of a bread product is one serving

Your dietitian can help you be more exact.

Cereals/Grains/Pasta

Bran cereals*, concentrated (such as Bran Buds®, All Bran®)	⅓ cup
Bran cereals, flaked	½ cup
Bulgur (cooked)	½ cup
Cooked cereals	½ cup
Cornmeal (dry)	2½ tablespoons
Grapenuts®	3 tablespoons
Grits (cooked)	½ cup
Other ready-to-eat unsweetened cereals	¾ cup
Pasta (cooked)	½ cup
Puffed cereal	1½ cups
Rice, white or brown (cooked)	⅓ cup
Shredded wheat	½ cup
Wheat germ*	3 tablespoons

Dried Beans, Peas/Lentils

Beans* and peas* (cooked), such as kidney, white, split, blackeye	⅓ cup
Baked beans*	¼ cup
Lentils* (cooked)	⅓ cup

Starchy Vegetables

Corn*	½ cup
Corn on cob, 6 inches long	1

* 3 grams or more of fiber per serving.

Lima beans*	½ cup
Peas, green* (canned or frozen)	½ cup
Plantain*	½ cup
Potato, baked	1 small (3 ounces)
Potato, mashed	½ cup
Squash, winter* (acorn, butternut)	¾ cup
Yam, sweet potato, plain	⅓ cup

Bread

Bagel	½ (1 ounce)
Bread sticks, crisp, 4 inches long x ½ inch wide	2 (⅔ ounce)
Croutons, lowfat	1 cup
English muffin	½
Frankfurter or hamburger bun	½ (1 ounce)
Pita, 6 inches across	½
Plain roll, small	1 (1 ounce)
Raisin, unfrosted	1 slice (1 ounce)
Rye*, pumpernickel*	1 slice (1 ounce)
Tortilla, 6 inches across	1
White (including French, Italian)	1 slice (1 ounce)
Whole wheat	1 slice (1 ounce)

Crackers/Snacks

Animal crackers	8
Graham crackers, 2½-inch square	3
Matzo	¾ ounce
Melba toast	5 slices
Oyster crackers	24
Popcorn (popped, no fat added)	3 cups
Pretzels	¾ ounce
Rye crisp, 2 inches x 3½ inches	4
Saltine-type crackers	6
Whole wheat crackers, no fat added (crisp breads, such as Finn®, Kavli®, Wasa®)	2–4 slices (¾ ounce)

Starch Foods Prepared with Fat
(Count as 1 starch/bread serving, plus 1 fat serving)

Biscuit, 2½ inches across	1
Chow mein noodles	½ cup
Corn bread, 2-inch cube	1 (2 ounces)

* 3 grams or more of fiber per serving.

Cracker, round butter type	6
French fried potatoes, 2 to 3½ inches long	10 (1½ ounces)
Muffin, plain, small	1
Pancake, 4 inches across	2
Stuffing, bread (prepared)	¼ cup
Taco shell, 6 inches across	2
Waffle, 4½-inch square	1
Whole wheat crackers, fat added (such as Triscuits®)	4–6 (1 ounce)

Meat List

Each serving of meat and substitutes on this list contains varying amounts of fat and calories. The list is divided into three parts based on the amount of fat and calories: lean meat, medium-fat meat, and high-fat meat. One ounce (one meat exchange) of each of these includes:

	Carbohydrate (grams)	Protein (grams)	Fat (grams)	Calories
Lean	0	7	3	55
Medium-Fat	0	7	5	75
High-Fat	0	7	8	100

You are encouraged to use more lean and medium-fat meat, poultry, and fish in your meal plan. This will help decrease your fat intake, which may help decrease your risk for heart disease. The items from the high-fat group are high in saturated fat, cholesterol, and calories. You should limit your choices from the high-fat group to three (3) times per week. Meat and substitutes do not contribute any fiber to your meal plan.

Tips:

- Bake, roast, broil, grill, or boil these foods rather than frying them with added fat.
- Use a nonstick pan spray or a nonstick pan to brown or fry these foods.
- Trim off visible fat before and after cooking.
- Do not add flour, bread crumbs, coating mixes, or fat to these foods when preparing them.
- Weigh meat after removing bones and fat, and after cooking. Three ounces

of cooked meat is about equal to 4 ounces of raw meat. Some examples of meat portions are:

2 ounces meat (2 meat exchanges	= 1 small chicken leg or thigh ½ cup cottage cheese or tuna
3 ounces meat (3 meat exchanges	= 1 medium pork chop 1 small hamburger ½ chicken breast (1 side) 1 unbreaded fish fillet cooked meat, about the size of a deck of cards

• Restaurants usually serve prime cuts of meat, which are high in fat and calories.

Lean Meat and Substitutes
(One exchange is equal to any one of the following items)

Beef:	USDA good or choice grades of lean beef, such as round, sirloin, flank steak, tenderloin, chipped beef*.	1 ounce
Pork:	Lean pork, such as fresh ham; canned, cured or boiled ham*; Canadian bacon*; tenderloin.	1 ounce
Veal:	All cuts are lean except for veal cutlets (ground or cubed). Examples of lean veal are chops and roasts.	1 ounce
Poultry:	Chicken, turkey, Cornish hen (without skin)	1 ounce
Fish:	All fresh and frozen fish	1 ounce
	Crab, lobster, scallops, shrimp, clams* (fresh, or canned in water)	1 ounce (¼ cup)
	Oysters	3 ounces (5 to 7 medium)
	Tuna* (canned in water)	¼ cup
	Herring (uncreamed or smoked)	1 ounce
	Sardines (canned)	2 medium
Wild Game:	Venison, rabbit, squirrel	1 ounce
	Pheasant, duck, goose (without skin)	1 ounce
Cheese:	Any cottage cheese	¼ cup
	Grated parmesan	2 tablespoons
	Diet cheeses* with less than 55 calories per ounce	1 ounce

* 400 mg or more of sodium per exchange.

Other:	95 percent fat-free luncheon meat*	1 ounce
	Egg whites	3 whites
	Egg substitutes with less than 55 calories per ¼ cup	¼ cup

Medium-Fat Meat and Substitutes
(One exchange is equal to any one of the following items)

Beef:	Most beef products fall into this category. Examples are: all ground beef, roast (rib, chuck, rump), steak (cubed, Porterhouse, T-bone), and meatloaf	1 ounce
Pork:	Most pork products fall into this category. Examples are: chops, loin roast, Boston butt, cutlets	1 ounce
Lamb:	Most lamb products fall into this category. Examples are: chops, leg, and roast.	1 ounce
Veal:	Cutlet (ground or cubed, unbreaded)	1 ounce
Poultry:	Chicken (with skin), domestic duck or goose (well-drained of fat), ground turkey	1 ounce
Fish:	Tuna* (canned in oil and drained), salmon* (canned)	¼ cup
Cheese:	Skim or part-skim milk cheeses, such as:	
	Ricotta	¼ cup
	Mozzarella	1 ounce
	Diet cheeses* with 56–80 calories per ounce	1 ounce
Other:	86 percent fat-free luncheon meat*	1 ounce
	Egg (high in cholesterol, limit to 3 per week)	1
	Egg substitutes with 56–80 calories per ¼ cup	¼ cup
	Tofu (2½ x 2¾ x 1 inches)	4 ounces
	Liver, heart, kidney, sweetbreads (high in cholesterol)	1 ounce

High-Fat Meat and Substitutes

Remember, these items are high in saturated fat, cholesterol, and calories, and should be used only three (3) times per week. One exchange is equal to any one of the following items.

| *Beef:* | Most USDA prime cuts of beef, such as ribs, corned beef* | 1 ounce |

* 400 mg or more of sodium per exchange.

Pork:	Spareribs, ground pork, pork sausage* (patty or link)	1 ounce
Lamb:	Patties (ground lamb)	1 ounce
Fish:	Any fried fish product	1 ounce
Cheese:	All regular cheeses*, such as American, Blue, Cheddar, Monterey, Swiss	1 ounce
Other:	Luncheon meat*, such as bologna, salami, pimento loaf	1 ounce
	Sausage*, such as Polish, Italian, knockwurst, smoked	1 ounce
	Bratwurst*	1 ounce
	Frankfurter* (turkey or chicken)	1 frank (10 per pound)
	Peanut Butter (contains unsaturated fat)	1 tablespoon

Count as one high-fat meat plus one fat exchange:

	Frankfurter* (beef, pork, or combination)	1 frank (10 per pound)

Vegetable List

Each vegetable serving on this list contains about 5 grams of carbohydrate, 2 grams of protein, and 25 calories. Vegetables contain 2–3 grams of dietary fiber.

Vegetables are a good source of vitamins and minerals. Fresh and frozen vegetables have more vitamins and less added salt. Rinsing canned vegetables will remove much of the salt.

Unless otherwise noted, the serving size for vegetables is:

- ½ cup of cooked vegetables or vegetable juice
- 1 cup of raw vegetables

Artichoke (½ medium)	Carrots	Okra
Asparagus	Cauliflower	Onions
Beans (green, wax, Italian)	Eggplant	Pea pods
Bean sprouts	Greens (collard, mustard, turnip)	Peppers (green)
Beets		Rutabaga
Broccoli	Kohlrabi	Sauerkraut*
Brussels sprouts	Leeks	Spinach, cooked
Cabbage, cooked	Mushrooms, cooked	Summer squash

* 400 mg or more of sodium per exchange.

(crookneck)	Tomato/vegetable juice*	Water chestnuts
Tomato (one large)	Turnips	Zucchini, cooked

Starchy vegetables such as corn, peas, and potatoes are found on the **Starch/Bread** list.

For free vegetables, see **Free Food** list on pages 204–206.

Fruit List

Each item on this list contains about 15 grams of carbohydrate, and 60 calories. Fresh, frozen, and dry fruits have about 2 grams of fiber per serving. Fruit juices contain very little dietary fiber.

The carbohydrate and calorie content for a fruit serving are based on the usual serving of the most commonly eaten fruits. Use fresh fruits, or fruits frozen or canned without sugar added. Whole fruit is more filling than fruit juice, and may be a better choice for those who are trying to lose weight. Unless otherwise noted, the serving size for fruit is:

- ½ cup of fresh fruit or fruit juice
- ¼ cup of dried fruit

Fresh, frozen, and unsweetened canned fruit

Apple (raw, 2 inches across)	1 apple
Applesauce (unsweetened)	½ cup
Apricots (medium, raw)	4 apricots
Apricots (canned)	½ cup, or 4 halves
Banana (9 inches long)	½ banana
Blackberries † (raw)	¾ cup
Blueberries † (raw)	¾ cup
Cantaloupe (5 inches across)	⅓ melon
cubes	1 cup
Cherries (large, sweet, raw)	12 cherries
Cherries (canned)	½ cup
Figs (raw, 2 inches across)	2 figs
Fruit cocktail (canned)	½ cup
Grapefruit (medium)	½ grapefruit
Grapefruit (segments)	¾ cup

* 400 mg or more of sodium per exchange.
† 3 or more grams of fiber per serving.

Grapes (small)	15 grapes
Honeydew melon (medium)	⅛ melon
cubes	1 cup
Kiwi (large)	1 kiwi
Mandarin oranges	¾ cup
Mango (small)	½ mango
Nectarine* (1½ inches across)	1 nectarine
Orange (2½ inches across)	1 orange
Papaya	1 cup
Peach (2¾ inches across)	1 peach, or ¾ cup
Peaches (canned)	½ cup, or 2 halves
Pear	½ large, 1 small
Pears (canned)	½ cup, or 2 halves
Persimmon (medium, native)	2 persimmons
Pineapple (raw)	¾ cup
Pineapple (canned)	⅓ cup
Plum (raw, 2 inches across)	2 plums
Pomegranate*	½ pomegranate
Raspberries* (raw)	1 cup
Strawberries* (raw, whole)	1¼ cup
Tangerine* (2½ inches across)	2 tangerines
Watermelon (cubes)	1¼ cups

Dried Fruit

Apples*	4 rings
Apricots*	7 halves
Dates	2½ medium
Figs*	1½
Prunes*	3 medium
Raisins	2 tablespoons

Fruit Juice

Apple juice/cider	½ cup
Cranberry juice cocktail	⅓ cup
Grapefruit juice	½ cup
Grape juice	⅓ cup
Orange juice	½ cup
Pineapple juice	½ cup
Prune juice	⅓ cup

* 3 or more grams of fiber per serving.

Milk List

E ach serving of milk or milk products on this list contains about 12 grams of carbohydrate and 8 grams of protein. The amount of fat in milk is measured in percent of butterfat. The calories vary, depending on what kind of milk you choose. The list is divided into three parts based on the amount of fat and calories: skim/very lowfat milk, lowfat milk, and whole milk. One serving (one milk exchange) of each of these includes:

	Carbohydrate (grams)	Protein (grams)	Fat (grams)	Calories
Skim/Very Lowfat	12	8	trace	90
Lowfat	12	8	5	120
Whole	12	8	8	150

Milk is the body's main source of calcium, the mineral needed for growth and repair of bones. Yogurt is also a good source of calcium. Yogurt and many dry or powdered milk products have different amounts of fat. If you have questions about a particular item, read the label to find out the fat and calorie content.

Milk is good to drink, but it can also be added to cereal, and to other foods. Many tasty dishes such as sugar-free pudding are made with milk. Plain yogurt is delicious with one of your fruit servings mixed with it.

Skim and Very Lowfat Milk

1 cup skim milk
1 cup ½ percent milk
1 cup 1 percent milk
1 cup lowfat buttermilk
½ cup evaporated skim milk
⅓ cup dry nonfat milk
8-ounce carton plain nonfat yogurt

Lowfat Milk

1 cup fluid 2 percent milk
8-ounce carton plain lowfat yogurt (with added nonfat milk solids)

Whole Milk

The whole milk group has much more fat per serving than the skim and lowfat groups. Whole milk has more than 3¼ percent butterfat. Try to limit your choices from the whole milk group as much as possible.

1 cup whole milk
½ cup evaporated whole milk
8-ounce carton whole plain yogurt

Fat List

E ach serving on the fat list contains about 5 grams of fat and 45 calories.
   The foods on the fat list contain mostly fat, although some items may also contain a small amount of protein. All fats are high in calories, and should be carefully measured. Everyone should modify fat intake by eating unsaturated fats instead of saturated fats. The sodium content of these foods varies widely. Check the label for sodium information.

Unsaturated Fats

Avocado	⅛ medium
Margarine	1 teaspoon
Margarine, diet*	1 tablespoon
Mayonnaise	1 teaspoon
Mayonnaise, reduced-calorie*	1 tablespoon
Nuts and Seeds:	
Almonds, dry roasted	6 whole
Cashews, dry roasted	1 tablespoon
Pecans	2 whole
Peanuts	20 small, 10 large
Walnuts	2 whole
Other nuts	1 tablespoon
Seeds, pine nuts, sunflower (without shells)	1 tablespoon
Pumpkin seeds	2 teaspoons

* If more than one or two servings are consumed, sodium levels will equal or exceed 400 mg.

Oil (corn, cottonseed, safflower, soybean, sunflower, olive, peanut)	1 teaspoon
Olives*	10 small, 5 large
Salad dressing, mayonnaise-type	2 teaspoons
Salad dressing, mayonnaise-type, reduced-calorie	1 tablespoon
Salad dressing (all varieties)*	1 tablespoon
Salad dressing, reduced-calorie†	2 tablespoons

(Two tablespoons of low-calorie salad dressing is a free food.)

Saturated Fats

Butter	1 teaspoon
Bacon*	1 slice
Chitterlings	½ ounce
Coconut, shredded	2 tablespoons
Coffee whitener, liquid	2 tablespoons
Coffee whitener, powder	4 teaspoons
Cream (light, coffee, table)	2 tablespoons
Cream, sour	2 tablespoons
Cream (heavy, whipping)	1 tablespoon
Cream cheese	1 tablespoon
Salt pork*	¼ ounce

Free Foods

A free food is any food or drink that contains 20 calories or less per serving. You can eat as much as you want of those items that have no serving size specified. You may eat two or three servings per day of those items that have a specific serving size. Be sure to spread them out through the day.

Drinks

Bouillon†, or broth without fat§
Bouillon, low-sodium
Carbonated drinks, sugar-free
Carbonated water

* If more than one or two servings are consumed, sodium levels will equal or exceed 400 mg.
† 400 mg or more of sodium per serving.
§ 3 grams or more of fiber per serving.

Club soda
Cocoa powder, unsweetened (1 tablespoon)
Coffee/Tea
Drink mixes, sugar-free
Mineral water
Tonic water, sugar-free

Nonstick pan spray

Fruit

Cranberries, unsweetened (½ cup)
Rhubarb, unsweetened (½ cup)

**Vegetables
(raw, 1 cup)**

Cabbage
Celery
Chinese cabbage*
Cucumber
Green onion
Hot peppers
Mushrooms
Radishes
Zucchini*
Salad greens:
    Endive
    Escarole
    Lettuce
    Romaine
    Spinach

Sweet Substitutes

Candy, hard, sugar-free
Gelatin, sugar-free
Gum, sugar-free
Jam/jelly, sugar-free (2 teaspoons)
Pancake syrup, sugar-free (¼ cup)
Sugar substitutes (saccharin, Equal)
Whipped topping, low-calorie

* 3 grams or more of fiber per serving.

Condiments

Catsup (1 tablespoon)
Horseradish
Mustard
Pickles*, dill, unsweetened
Salad dressing, low-calorie (2 tablespoons)
Taco sauce (1 tablespoon)

Seasonings can be very helpful in making food taste better. Be careful of how much sodium you use. Read the label, and choose seasonings that do not contain sodium or salt.

Basil (fresh)
Celery seeds
Cinnamon
Chili powder
Chives
Curry
Dill
Flavoring extracts (vanilla, lemon, almond, walnut, peppermint, butter, and the like)

Garlic
Garlic powder
Herbs
Hot pepper sauce
Lemon
Lemon juice
Lemon pepper
Lime
Lime juice
Mint

Onion powder
Oregano
Paprika
Pepper
Pimento
Spices
Soy sauce*
Soy sauce, low sodium
Wine, used in cooking (¼ cup)
Worcestershire sauce

* 400 mg or more of sodium per serving.

Appendix A

Conversion Tables for Metric Measurements

Liquid Measures

[1 liter = 10 deciliters (dl) = 100 centiliters (cl) = 1,000 milliliters (ml)]

Spoons, cups, pints, and quarts	Liquid ounces	Metric equivalent
1 tsp	¹⁄₁₆ oz	½ cl; 5 ml
1 Tb	½ oz	15 ml
¼ c; 4 Tb	2 oz	½ dl; 59 ml
⅓ c; 5 Tb	2⅔ oz	¾ dl; 79 ml
½ c	4 oz	1 dl; 119 ml
1 c	8 oz	¼ l; 237 ml
1¼ c	10 oz	3 dl; 296 ml
2 c; 1 pt	16 oz	½ l; 473 ml
2½ c	20 oz	592 ml
3 c	24 oz	710 ml; ¾ l
4 c; 1 qt	32 oz	1 l; 946 ml
4 qt; 1 gal	128 oz	3¾ l; 3,785 ml
5 qt		4¾ l
6 qt		5¾ l
8 qt		7½ l

Conversion formula: To convert liters to quarts, multiply the liters by .95; quarts to liters, multiply the quarts by 1.057.

Source: From *The Joy of Microwaving,* published by Prentice Hall Press, 1986.

Weight

American ounces	American pounds	Grams	Kilograms
⅓ oz		10 g	
½ oz		15 g	
1 oz		30 g	
3½ oz		100 g	
4 oz	¼ lb	114 g	
5 oz		140 g	
8 oz	½ lb	227 g	
9 oz		250 g	¼ kg
16 oz	1 lb	450 g	
18 oz	1⅛ lb	500 g	½ kg
32 oz	2 lb	900 g	
36 oz	2¼ lb	1000 g	1 kg
	3 lb	1350 g	1⅓ kg
	4 lb	2800 g	1¾ kg

Conversion formula: To convert ounces into grams, multiply the ounces by 28.35; grams into ounces, multiply the grams by .035.

Source: From *The Joy of Microwaving,* published by Prentice Hall Press, 1986.

Appendix B

Temperature Conversion Table
Temperatures

Fahrenheit	Celsius
32° *	0°
60°	16°
75°	24°
80°	27°
95°	37°
150°	65°
175°	79°
212° †	100°
250°	121°
300°	149°
350°	177°
400°	205°
450°	232°
500°	260°

* water freezes
† water boils
Conversion formula: To convert Fahrenheit into Celsius, subtract 32, multiply by 5, divide by 9. To convert Celsius to Fahrenheit, multiply by 9, divide by 5, add 32.
Source: From *The Joy of Microwaving,* published by Prentice Hall Press, 1986.

Index

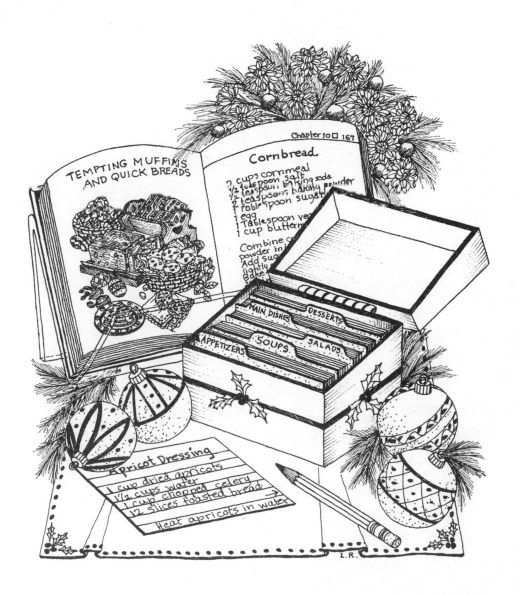

A

Acorn squash
  acorn squash soup, 63
  cranberry-stuffed acorn squash, 75
Adjusting favorite recipes, 9–16
Alcohol, 5
Appetizers
  baked shrimp scampi, 35
  barbecued prawns, 32
  broiled herbed scallops, 34
  broiled mushroom caps, 37
  cherry tomatoes with crab, 39
  cherry tomatoes with pesto filling, 29
  marinated crayfish tails, 32
  Moroccan dip, 31
  oysters casino, 40
  pears with ricotta, 38
  potato hors d'oeuvres, 36
  ricotta cassata, 33
  salmon dip, 31
  sapsago cheese rolls, 30
  steamed mussels, 35
  tasty stuffed mushrooms, 37
Apples
  apple and prune dressing, 91
  baked apples with raisins, 79
  low-calorie apple dressing, 85
Apricots
  apricot dressing for turkey, 92
  apricot kolachy, 106
  apricot muffins, 138

B

Banana bread, 144
Beet salad, sliced, 52
Beverages, 27–46
  Christmas cranberry punch, 46
  cranberry cooler, 43
  fruit punch, 44
  hot wassail, 45
  kiwi-yogurt smoothie, 42
  low-calorie eggnog, 45
  Merry cranberry punch, 41
  raspberry smoothie, 42
  spicy tomato cocktail, 44
  tomato cocktail, 43
Blueberry muffins, 13–14
Bran
  bran muffins, 133
  peanut butter-bran muffins, 133
Bread exchanges, 194–196
Breads, *see also* Muffins and Quick breads, Yeast breads and yeast cakes
  Challah (holiday twist bread), 183
  mandelbrot (almond bread), 182
Broccoli soup, purée of, 59
Brussels sprouts with walnuts, 76
Buttermilk pancakes, 15–16
Butternut squash with ginger, 74

C

Cabbage soup, 61
Cakes/fruitcakes
  fruitcake, 151
  honey cake, 184
  pumpkin fruitcake, 152
  thyme-fig fruitcake, 153
Calories, 3
Carbohydrates, 4
Carrots
  carrot cake muffin treats, 139
  pineapple-carrot coffee ring, 117
Casseroles
  African vegetable stew, 95
  cheese and rice casserole, 99
  eggplant-Swiss cheese casserole, 100
  rice and lentils, 93
  tofu fiesta, 94
Cauliflower
  cauliflower piquante, 77
  fresh cauliflower salad, 54
Cherry tomatoes
  cherry tomatoes with crab, 37
  cherry tomatoes with pesto filling, 29
  Chicken-rice soup, 65
Christmas menus, 21–23
Cookies, *see* Desserts
Corn muffins, 136
Crab, cherry tomatoes with, 39
Cranberries
  Christmas cranberry punch, 46
  cranberry cooler, 43
  cranberry-nut bread, 146
  cranberry-orange bars, 126
  cranberry-orange muffins, 135
  cranberry-raisin sauce, 78
  cranberry relish, 56
  cranberry-rice stuffing, 88
  cranberry-stuffed acorn squash, 75
  cranberry sweet potatoes, 79
  cranberry-wild rice stuffing, 90
  holiday cranberry rolls, 110
  Merry cranberry punch, 41
Crayfish, marinated, 32
Cucumber salad, 55

D

Desserts
  applesauce-raisin cookies, 124
  Christmas fruitcake cookies, 125
  cranberry-orange bars, 126
  fruit and nut balls, 123
  prune-coconut bars, 128
  pumpkin-oatmeal bars, 127
  raisin bars, 129
  rolled sugar cookies, 130
  Russian tea cakes, 123
Diet therapy for diabetes, 6–7
Disaccharides, 4
Dressing/stuffing
  apple and prune dressing, 91
  apricot dressing for turkey, 92
  bread stuffing, 86
  corn bread stuffing, 85
  cranberry-rice stuffing, 88
  cranberry-wild rice stuffing, 90
  low-calorie apple dressing, 85
  pecan corn bread stuffing, 86
  traditional bread dressing, 87
  wild rice-pine nut stuffing, 89

E

Eggnog, low-calorie, 45
Eggplant-Swiss cheese casserole, 100
Exercise and diabetes, 5, 6

F

Fat exchanges, 203–204
Fats and high-fat foods, 3–4
Fiber, 4
Fig square, 107
Food exchanges, using, 191–193
Fruit
    baked apples with raisins, 79
    fresh fruit ambrosia, 81
Fruit exchanges, 200–201
Fruitcake, 151; *see also* Cakes/ fruitcakes

G

Glucose, 5

H

Hearts of Palm salad, 53
Hors d'oeuvres, potato, 36

I

Insulin, 5
Insulin resistance, 5–6

J

Jewish recipes
    baked gefilte fish, 181
    beef cholent, 175
    gefilte fish, 179
    honey cake, 184
    Kaese blintzes (rolled cheese pancakes), 185
    lamb and brown rice pilaf, 178
    Latkes, 176
    Lokshen Kugel (noodle pudding), 186
    mandelbrot, 182
    meaty split pea soup, 186
    sweet and sour green beans, 187
    Tzimmes, 180
    Zimsterne, 177

K

Kiwi
    kiwi-tomato salad, 49
    kiwi-yogurt smoothie, 42

L

Lacto-Ovo
  Christmas menus, 21–22
  New Year's menus, 24
  Thanksgiving menus, 20
Lamb and brown rice pilaf, 178
Lentils
  hearty lentil soup, 66
  lentil salad, 51
  rice and lentils, 93

M

Meat exchanges, 196–199
Menus, 17–26
Milk/dairy food(s) exchange(s), 202–203
Monosaccharides, 4
Muffins and quick breads
  apricot muffins, 138
  baking powder biscuits, 140
  banana bread, 144
  blueberry muffins, 13–14
  bran muffins, 133
  carrot cake muffin treats, 139
  corn bread, 143
  corn muffins, 136
  cranberry-nut bread, 146
  cranberry-orange muffins, 135
  dilly rice muffins, 137
  low-cholesterol popovers, 141
  oatmeal-banana muffins, 134
  peanut butter-bran muffins, 133
  pumpkin-bran muffins, 140
  pumpkin pancakes, 141
  pumpkin-raisin bread, 145
  pumpkin-raisin muffins, 136
  whole wheat-buttermilk pancakes, 142
Mushrooms
  broiled mushroom caps, 37
  tasty stuffed mushrooms, 37
Mussels, steamed, 35

N

New Year's menus, 23–25
Nutrients, 3
Nutrition and diabetes, 5–7

O

Oatmeal
  oatmeal-banana muffins, 134
  oatmeal-bran bread, 112
Onion soup, 64
Oranges
  cranberry-orange muffins, 135
  orange waldorf salad, 53
  sweet potatoes a l'orange, 80
  zesty orange salad, 52
Oysters
  oyster stew, 67
  oysters casino, 40

P

Pancakes
    adjusting favorite recipes for, 15–16
    buttermilk pancakes, 15
    Kaese blintzes (rolled cheese pancakes), 185
    potato pancakes, 176
    pumpkin pancakes, 141
    sauces for, 147
    whole wheat-buttermilk pancakes, 142
Passover Seder meal, 25
Peanut butter
    peanut butter-bran muffins, 133
    peanut butter cookies, 11–12
Pears
    pear tea ring, 116
    pears with ricotta, 38
Pickled beets, 80
Pineapple
    molded turkey-pineapple salad, 164
    pineapple-carrot coffee ring, 117
Pizza
    brunch pizza, 98
    stuffed cheese pizza, 96
    whole wheat pizza, 97
Polysaccharides, 4
Potatoes
    oven-baked herbed potatoes, 78
    potato hors d'oeuvres, 36
    potato pancakes, 176
    savory potato soup, 160
Prawns, barbecued, 32
Prune-coconut bars, 128

Pumpkin
    baked stuffed pumpkin, 76
    pumpkin-bran muffins, 140
    pumpkin fruitcake, 152
    pumpkin-oatmeal bars, 127
    pumpkin pancakes, 141
    pumpkin-raisin bread, 145
    pumpkin-raisin muffins, 136
    pumpkin tea ring, 105
Punch
    Christmas cranberry punch, 46
    fruit punch, 44
    Merry cranberry punch, 41

R

Raspberry smoothie, 42
Ratatouille, 71
Relishes
    cranapple relish, 57
    cranberry relish, 56
Ricotta
    pears with ricotta, 38
    ricotta cassatta, 33
Rosh Hashanah dinner menu, 25

S

Sabbath meal-in-one, 175
Sabbath meal menu, 26
Saffron bread, 108

Salad dressings
    creamy garlic dressing, 59
    Dijon mustard dressing, 58
    French dressing, 57
    fresh Italian dressing, 58
Salads
    cucumber salad, 55
    Dijon-broccoli salad, 50
    four-bean salad, 50
    fresh cauliflower salad, 54
    hearts of palm salad, 53
    kiwi-tomato salad, 49
    lentil salad, 57
    orange waldorf salad, 53
    sliced beet salad, 52
    traditional waldorf salad, 49
    wild rice waldorf salad, 56
    zesty orange salad, 52
Salmon dip, 31
Sapsago cheese rolls, 30
Sauces
    cranberry-raisin sauce, 78
    fruit sauce for pancakes, 147
    rum-flavored fruit sauce, 147
Scallops, broiled herbed, 34
Scampi, baked, 35
Soups
    acorn squash soup, 63
    cabbage soup, 61
    chicken-rice soup, 65
    green split pea soup, 67
    hearty lentil soup, 66
    low-calorie minestrone, 61
    meaty split pea soup, 186
    onion soup, 64
    oyster stew, 67
    purée of broccoli soup, 59
    savory potato soup, 60
    tomato-shrimp chowder, 62
    vegetable-barley soup, 60

Spicy star cookies, 177
Stress, and diabetes, 5
Stuffing, *see* Dressing/stuffing

T

Taco salad with cumin dressing,
    157
Thanksgiving menus, 19–20
Tofu fiesta, 94
Tomatoes
    tomato cocktail, 43
    spicy tomato cocktail, 44
    tomato-shrimp chowder, 62
Turkey recipes for leftovers
    curried turkey on rice, 159
    curry turkey stir-fry, 160
    Hawaiian turkey kebobs, 162
    molded turkey-pineapple salad,
        164
    Shepherd's turkey pie, 158
    spicy rice pilaf with turkey, 169
    taco salad with cumin dressing,
        157
    turkey barbecue for sandwiches,
        170
    turkey-barley soup, 168
    turkey chili, 167
    turkey chowder, 166
    turkey frittata, 172
    turkey gumbo, 163
    turkey-orange salad, 160
    turkey spaghetti sauce, 171
    turkey-spinach lasagna, 165
    wild rice-turkey salad, 161
Type I diabetes, 5
Type II diabetes, 5–6

V

Variety in diet, 3
Vegetable exchanges, 199–200
Vegetables
  baked stuffed pumpkin, 77
  baked zucchini with cheese, 76
  brussels sprouts with walnuts, 76
  butternut squash with ginger, 74
  cauliflower piquante, 77
  cranberry-stuffed acorn squash, 75
  cranberry sweet potatoes, 79
  fennel and rice, 73
  Italian steamed artichokes, 72
  oven-baked herbed potatoes, 78
  ratatouille, 71
  sweet and sour green beans, 187
  sweet potatoes a l'orange, 80
  vegetable confetti, 73
  wild rice-stuffed squash, 74
  zucchini mandarin, 71
Vegetarian menus
  Christmas menus, 22–23
  New Year's menus, 24–25
  Thanksgiving menus, 20

W

Weight reduction, and diabetes, 6
Wild rice
  cranberry-wild rice stuffing, 90
  wild rice-pine nut stuffing, 89
  wild rice-stuffed squash, 74
  wild rice-turkey salad, 161

Y

Yeast, measurement of, 101
Yeast breads and yeast cakes
  apricot kolachy, 106
  Christmas stollen, 104
  fig square, 107
  Greek Christmas bread, 113
  holiday cranberry rolls, 110
  holiday fruit and nut bread, 115
  no-knead bran bread, 118
  oatmeal-bran bread, 112
  pear tea ring, 116
  pineapple carrot coffee ring,
    117
  pumpkin tea ring, 105
  saffron bread, 108
  Swedish cardamom braid, 109
  Swedish tea log, 103
  whole wheat bread, 119
  whole wheat-pecan rolls, 111
  Yugoslavian Christmas bread
    "Potika," 114

Z

Zucchini, baked with cheese, 76